Klaus Dieter Maria Resch

Transendoscopic Ultrasound
for Neurosurgery

Klaus Dieter Maria Resch

Transendoscopic Ultrasound for Neurosurgery

With 257 Figures, 150 in Color
and 11 Tables

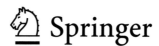

Klaus Dieter Maria Resch, M. D.
Universitätsklinikum Greifswald
Klinik und Poliklinik für Neurochirurgie
Sauerbruchstraße 1
17487 Greifswald, Germany

Library of Congress Control Number: 2005924217

ISBN-10 3-540-42505-5
Springer Berlin Heidelberg New York
ISBN-13 978-3-540-42505-2
Springer Berlin Heidelberg New York

Springer is a part of Springer Science + Business Media
springeronline.com
© Springer-Verlag Berlin Heidelberg 2006
Printed in Germany

Editor: Gabriele Schröder, 69121 Heidelberg, Germany
Desk Editor: Stephanie Benko, 69121 Heidelberg, Germany
Production: ProEdit GmbH, 69126 Heidelberg, Germany
Cover design: Frido Steinen-Broo, eStudio Calamar, Pau/Girona, Spain
Typesetting and reproduction of the figures: AM-productions GmbH, 69168 Wiesloch, Germany

Printed on acid-free paper   24/3151 ML   5 4 3 2 1 0

To the Reader

This book is not intended for easy reading, but is written for those who want to familiarize themselves with a new method of intraoperative imaging and a navigation tool in neuroendoscopy. Therefore, it starts with numerous laboratory cases, since it is the strong opinion of the author that it is only after gaining sufficient laboratory experience that the specialist can be sufficiently competent in applying this new method in the operating room.

It might be quite tempting to try out this new method prematurely, but it is unsuitable for learning 'by doing' or by 'trial and error.' Therefore, only prior knowledge of a sufficient number of 'landmarks' will enhance the professional's 'insight,' and this can easily be achieved in the laboratory, or at least by an ENS course (www.ens-surgery.com, link: ENS-course). Only then can this new tool be fully employed to let us reach beyond the current boundaries of our expertise. For the result-oriented reader, however, the major focus of interest will be in the third chapter of the book: "*Clinical Cases*".

The content of this book was compiled by the author between 1996 and 2002 at the university clinics of Mainz, Dresden, and Greifswald and at the Institute of Anatomy and Cell Biology at the University of Heidelberg.

Special credit is due to Prof. Dr. G. Schackert in Dresden, who agreed to complete the clinical series previously started in Mainz. Major credit also goes to Prof. Dr. A. Perneczky for his willingness to support this project exploiting previously uncharted territory; after his initial strong support overriding priorities compelled him to hand on the project to the present author. Prof. Dr. W. Kriz and Prof. Dr. K. Tiedemann supported the project by hosting consecutive ENS courses.

My special thanks go to Messrs. ALOKA (Tokyo, Japan) and Messrs. R. Wolf (Knittlingen, Germany) for technical support and for providing the necessary equipment.

Finally, I cannot omit to acknowledge the helpful assistance of all those who have contributed to the realization of this project, and especially Mrs. Heide Roesler (www.creativeartservice.de), who patiently prepared the sophisticated computer graphics and the cover design for the book. Special thanks also go to Dr. Otto R. Maas and Dr. Andrew Alcock for reviewing the draft and making numerous valuable suggestions on the proper presentation of the subject.

Greifswald,   KLAUS DIETER MARIA RESCH
September 2005

Foreword

Neuroendoscopy has been a real revolution in the treatment of several disorders of the central nervous system. In the treatment of obstructive hydrocephalus and intracranial cystic lesions, above all, almost every surgeon has been somehow obliged to deal with the neuroendoscopic tools since the second half of the 1990s. The diffusion of the knowledge has been so rapid that the treatment of some well-defined conditions with techniques other than neuroendoscopy could now appear almost unnatural, especially to the younger generation of neurosurgeons who completed their training during the past 10 years. The images offered by the neuroendoscopes are fascinating because they show the pathology as it is, within the crystal-clear medium that is the natural environment of the brain cavities. The power of definition of the optic has been excellent from the very beginning with the rigid rod lenses systems, and the technology of cameras has allowed a growing power of resolution. Nevertheless, nothing so far could allow the surgeon to see what was hidden behind the anatomical structures so well visualized by the optics. In patients with significant distortion of the anatomy, such as large arachnoid cysts or multiloculated hydrocephalus, it can be easy to loose the orientation even for experienced neuroendoscopists. The target of the procedure, that often looks like a very thin membrane on pre-operative MRI, can reveal itself as a thick, whitish wall that limits the possibilities of the surgeon and increases the risks and the time of the procedure. Even in the most straightforward procedure of neuroendoscopy, third ventriculostomy, sometimes the anatomy of the third ventricle floor can be surprisingly difficult to recognize, e.g. in the presence of associated central nervous system malformations or in patients presenting with shunt malfunction.

In all these cases, the possibility of "looking through" the membranes can really make the difference between a technical failure and a success. More importantly, it can significantly reduce the risks of the procedure, allowing the surgeon to choose a safer place for perforation of the membrane or helping him/her to understand the anatomy. Considering all this, the technique of endoneurosonography as described, improved and diffused by the author of this book really offers something valuable, the possibility of intra-operative imaging that is potentially more reliable, easier to use and less time consuming than the pre-operative imaging offered by pre-planning MRI performed for neuronavigation. In some cases the surgeon has to decide a very precise point where to coagulate and perforate a membrane, often only a few square millimeters in size. In these cases, intra-operative imaging can be invaluable. In common with all imaging techniques, good training is necessary for interpretation of intra-operative images. During surgery, especially in neuroendoscopy, the images obtained should be of good quality and rapidly understood by the surgeon, to avoid loss of time or performance of dangerous maneuvers only to obtain better images. Under this aspect, both the training courses in endoneurosonography organized by the author and this beautiful book are extremely welcome and will have an important impact in the rapidly progressing world of neuroendoscopy.

Giuseppe Cinalli
Head, Unit of Neuroendoscopy
Department of Pediatric Neurosurgery
Santobono Children's Hospital
via Mario Fiore n.6
80129 Naples, Italy
Tel. 39 081 2205762
Fax 39 081 2205660
Cell 39 335 6845214
e-mail: giuseppe.cinalli@fastwebnet.it

Contents

5 Future Concepts for Minimally Invasive Techniques in Neurosurgery

Chapter 1

Basics and Evolution of Endoneurosurgery

1

Contents

Introduction

The step from microneurosurgery to endoneurosurgery has meant a change to a minimally invasive technique, but at the same time the new technique is less safe (Schroeder et al. 1999), which limits its applicability. Further development have therefore had to be aimed at making neuroendoscopy safer. The current concept used to establish a near-real-time guidance system has involved the use of MR or CT, requiring enormous financial investment and technical effort (Albert et al. 1998; Black and Mehta 2000; Fahlbusch and Nimsky 2000; Grönemeyer et al. 1994; Hayashi et al. 1995; Kobayashi and Okudera 2000; Maciunas 1993; Wirtz et al. 2000). It is still not clear what surgical benefit this approach will have (Kelly 2000; Maciunas 2000; Paleologos et al. 2000; Shekhar 2000).

Another idea, therefore, was to equip the endoscope with a sonographic guidance system. As it stands, endoneurosonography is now a technique that can make a huge contribution to the elaboration of minimally invasive techniques in neurosurgery, as described below.

Evolution of Neurosurgery

Endoneurosonography was developed in a particular historical and technical environment and belongs to a recent phase of neurosurgical evolution. Retrospectively, the evolution of neurosurgery can be seen in steps, most of which are named after the underlying technical advances.

Neurosurgical phases by technical environment	
Cranial surgery (E. von Bergmann, E.T. Kocher, F. Krause, H. Cushing)	⇒ Neurosurgery
NC-OR within surgery (H. Cushing, O. Förster, W. Penfield)	⇒ NC-OR within neurosciences
NC-OR within neurosciences (R.W. Rand, L.I. Malis, M.G. Yasargil)	⇒ NC-OR within neuro- techniques
NC-OR within neurotechniques (A. Perneczky, M. Apuzzo)	⇒ NC-OR within high-tech medicine

The evolution of a new development always starts with a new idea, or a new vision, which is followed by a new concept; thus, it breaks previously uncharted ground, while still building step by step on past experience. All the threads of neurosurgery are still running side by side, even today. According to the paradigm theory of the history of science, evolution is not just always in progress; there is also change from one generation to the next. This is driven by aggressive competition between concepts and schools of thought (Kuhn 1969).

Neurosurgical phases by concept

1900 NC = surgery
(T. Billroth, E. von Bergmann, F. Durante, A. Chipault)

1930 Macro – NC
(F. Krause, O. Förster, V. Horsley, H. Cushing, etc.)

1970 Micro – NC
(R. W. Rand, L. I. Malis, M. G. Yasargil, etc.)

1990 MIN – NC
(A. Perneczky, T. Fukushima, K. Manwaring, etc.)

2000 High-tech – NC
(A. Perneczky, M. Apuzzo, M. Samii, etc.)

It is not yet clear whether the principles behind minimally invasive techniques (Cohen and Haines 1995; Fukuschima 1978; Perneczky 1999) and the image-guided and computer-assisted techniques (Black et al. 1997; Grönemeyer and Lufkin 2001; Maciunas 1993) are leading to parallel or diverging developments in neurosurgery.

These techniques are generally also used in combination and can be subsumed under the same headings (Galloway et al. 1993). Ideally, different techniques would be combined in such a way as to ensure that each will compensate for the side effects of the others. This is the ultimate goal of endoscopy-assisted microsurgery and endoneurosonography.

The concept of microsurgery, which does not only relate to the use of microtechniques, but also to application of the keyhole concept, was followed by the introduction of minimally invasive techniques into neurosurgery, which does not just mean using an endoscope rather than applying planning strategies. Surprisingly, this development went hand in hand with the advent of costly and bulky machines for intraoperative imaging or neuronavigation (Kikinis et al. 1996, 1998).

The main principle underlying microsurgery and keyhole surgery is 'nihil nocere' (do not harm) ideal of Hippocrates (Perneczky et al. 1999; Yasargil 1994a), and it is necessary to recognize that current methods of surgery do have to hurt for their target to be achieved. In neuroanatomy and neurophysiology, we have to cultivate enthusiasm for minimizing the trauma of surgery and of the surgical approach. This actually means that the subarachnoid approach should be selected as a natural anatomical pathway to the lesion (Yasargil 1984a, b) and that any trauma should be minimized to keep the homeostasis of the patient's brain, body, and mind intact (Yasargil 1994a–c).

Image-guided neurosurgery seems to change this concept in some way (Black et al. 1997; Kelly 2000; Kikinis et al. 1998; Maciunas 1993; Schlöndorf 1998; van Roost et al. 2001; Weinberg 1992; Wurm et al. 2000).

Imaging of Individual Anatomy

One of the strongest promoters of actual neurosurgery has been the evolution of imaging techniques. It is now possible to demonstrate the individual anatomy and pathoanatomy of any patient noninvasively. It is no longer necessary to open the patient up and then to see what can be done; a precise analysis of the individual situation is now possible (Perneczky 1992).

However, as a result of mathematical calculations, neuroradiological images have a different optical grammar than do natural images (Edelman 1992; ; Sacks 1989a, b; Weizäcker 1950).

There is a difference between visualization by optical means and images obtained by digital techniques. Von Weizäcker (1950) described the visual process in his book *Gestaltkreis*: "The optical apparatus and the CNS do not have a mathematical image of the space; indeed it forms the reality of space online." Digital media separate software and hardware, but the brain can deal with both together, being ruled by an evolutionary context (Poggio 1987). Any attempt to get a computer to see will reveal that viewing is a complex information processing task (Cooper and Shepard 1987; Gillam 1987, p. 109; Regan et al. 1987; Roth 1999). From a neurobiological point of view, visualization is a learning process of recognition (Edelmann 1992).

Planning an Individual Approach

Logically, for imaging of a patient's individual anatomy and the lesion suspected or known to be present an individual approach needs to be planned. Computer-assisted systems were used to reconstruct 3D images in elective approaches to simulate surgical strategies ahead of time (Kockro et al. 1999, 2000). These systems did not apply the neuroradiological findings in the operative field, however. In addition, the difference between digital imaging and optical visualization means that the information to be supplied to the neurosurgeon needs to have special characteristics to make the planning process comprehensible.

As a result of mathematical processing, digital imaging ends up in a world of pixels and voxels. During a surgical operation, or on endoneurosonography, visualization becomes possible as a result of neuronal processing and training, both of which involve 'biological coordinates,' such as:
- 3D system of the vascular tree
- Sulcogyral system
- Cisternal space system
- Ventricular cavity system
- Dural cover system
- Endoscopic landmarks (fingerprint system)
- Color-coding system
  (gray and white matter, tumor changes, etc.)
- Recording of locomotion
  (pulsation, shifting, CSF flow)
- Haptic feedback (mechanical behavior of tissue)

The sum of these biological coordinates creates neuropsychological feedback, which is superior to any monitoring with technical instruments. It therefore seems ridiculous to try to do this by technical means. The goal of monitoring and imaging must be to complement the biological feedback while presenting only such data as are required for neuropsychological feedback, such as:
- Real-time scan imaging of tissue (sonography)
- Imaging of fiber pathways and nuclei
  of the brain tissue
- Neurophysiological monitoring

Intelligent integration of these biological and technical recording and operant processes will be decisive when the following problems have to be faced:

Orientation Problem. In the past, planning and simulation were hampered in attempts to solve the orientation problem. Therefore, so-called navigation systems were developed, and these were readily accepted. However, it is not clear whether there is any benefit to the patient (Kelly 2000; Levy 1998; Maciunas 2000; Shekar 2000; Wirtz et al. 1997). Besides the financial, logistical, and ergonomic problems inherent in them, neuronavigation systems are lacking some characteristics that are important for orientation:
- Real-time capacity
- Ability to use biological coordinates (Resch 2002)
- Compatibility with neuropsychological needs
  of the surgeon's brain (Linke 1993, 1997, 1999)

Real-time Problem. The real-time problem does not just affect actual imaging, but also the understanding of complex imaging in the course of surgical decision making. It is a problem of information ergonomics, which will have to be solved by interface design.

The real-time capacity of imaging depends on the speed of the biological process (pulsation, CSF flow, bleeding, operative interaction, etc.) that has to be imaged. Of course, the best real-time characteristic at present is optical visualization. All imaging techniques must be evaluated against this standard.

Navigation Problem. Navigation in a biological space is not just a mathematical problem, but depends on (biological) tissue changes during surgery. Such changes might be:
- Shift of tissue
  (CSF, resection volume, spatula, etc.)
- Pathologic changes to anatomy and physiology
- Change in imaging characteristics
  of tissue during surgery
- Ergonomic changes with operational technique
  and environment

A technical system that ignores the biology of the field of application is never acceptable in a biological space.

Example: Navigation systems will present several possible transcerebral routes to reach the mediotemporal area (uncus, amygdala, etc.) from the temporal direction. However, the biology of the brain makes a subfrontal subarachnoidal (transcisternal) route advisable.

Neuronavigation is not just concerned with the problem of how to guide the instruments from one target to another, this being merely the object. The tools are only one part of the problem. The complex part of the problem is the process of navigation in the surgeon's brain and the interaction with the tools. For example, Linke (1997) remarks: "To use data from cognitive neuroscience for the theory and practice of neuronavigation is promising for the optimization of technical and didactic aspects of operating room techniques." The design of the interface between neuronavigation tools and surgeon will define the competence of such systems in the future. To be fully acceptable the navigation tool must allow intuitive use by the surgeon. This is well accepted in many fields in which safety standards are high (such as the joystick principle in the air force) (see chap. 5).

Technical Solution Steps

Historically, there are several approaches to the orientation problem, which are still current and necessary today:

- Topological neurology
  (fourth dimension, highly functional accuracy)
- Invasive imaging (angiography, encephalography, myelography, etc.)
- Noninvasive imaging (CT, MR)
- Sonography (pediatric, transfontanel)
- Computer-assisted planning and simulation systems
- Neuronavigation (without real-time imaging)
- Intraoperative imaging
  (CT/MR, near-real-time imaging)
- Intraoperative sonography
  (intraoperative real-time imaging)
- Intraoperative monitoring
  (physiological parameters)
- Functional imaging and image fusion
  (still a research tool)

In the evolution of the technical steps necessary one problem emerged as the most important: that of ergonomics in neurosurgery (Figs. 1.1, 1.2; see also chap. 5).

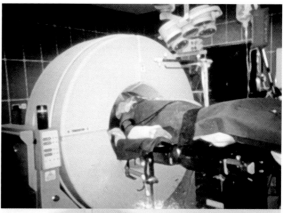

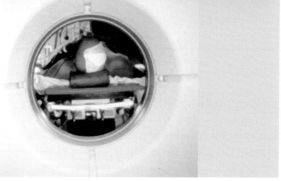

Fig. 1.1. Intraoperative CT. A mobile gantry for intraoperative CT imaging is shown. The patient on the operation table is not moved, but the CT scanner can be moved. Navigation and stereotaxy can be planned. Direct preoperative or postoperative imaging is feasible. Especially intraoperative imaging causes a problem of ergonomics in the OR.

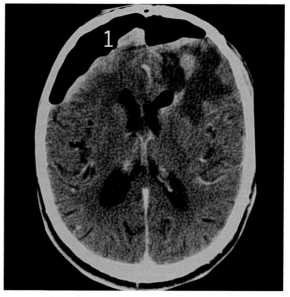

Fig. 1.2. Shift of tissue. Intraoperative CT imaging reveals a shift as a result of tumor resection and CSF release. The extent of intraoperative shift was surprisingly large as realized in the first cases in which the technique was applied

Ergonomic Problems in Neurosurgery

Examples of Ergonomic studies in neurosurgery are rare and are mostly limited to details (Al-Mefty 1989; Nunez and Kaufman 1988; Perneczky et al. 1999; Yasargil 1969). The goal of a minimally invasive concept in neurosurgery is to minimize the trauma to the brain and that caused by the approach with the aid of modern techniques and new concepts (Perneczky 1992; Perneczky et al. 1993, 1999). These techniques still have side effects:

■ Position of patient's head relative to the surgeon
Arrangements around the operation table often appear to be poorly coordinated, and a large number of instruments and several kinds of apparatus do not make for smooth operation and coordination of working procedures. This cannot be solved by design only, but rather requires neuropsychological discipline. The main intention has to be to avoid upsetting the ergonomics of the system 'patient and neurosurgeon' (Al-Mefty 1989; Patkin 1977, 1981; Yasargil 1994c, Resch 1999, 2002). The relation between the neurosurgeon's position and the position of the patient's head is a sensitive one that is often impaired, and then the surgeon's art seems to be handicapped, as ergonomic considerations are left out of play. This fact is appreciated by and well known to experienced neurosurgeons (Chandler 2000; Kelly 2000; Maciunas 2000; Shekhar 2000), but is not generally accepted (Paleologos et al. 2000).
New kinds of surgical instruments are now coming up (Cristante 2000). However, the large machines mentioned above (intraoperative CT, MR, neuronavigation systems) are trendy and prestigious (Apuzzo 1992, 1996; Kikinis et al. 1996, 1998; Steinmeier et al. 1998; Tronnier et al. 1998; Wirtz and Kunze 1998). It seems necessary to introduce the term 'ergonomic trauma,' which is something the patient may be subjected to (Resch 1999).

■ Miniaturization
In keeping with anatomy and physiology, there is no doubt that we will see advantages in miniaturization in the future. At present, however, it seems that this development has broken down. All components will have to be integrated smoothly, and the microtechnique must evolve to a 'microsystem technique' for ergonomic conditions to be achieved. From a scientific point of view, it does not make much sense to use a microscope in a macroscopic approach or to use an endoscope in a macroscopic or microsurgical approach. Endoscopically assisted microsurgery can be an interim solution, and the microscope will have to be replaced by the endoscope for many purposes (Cappabianca et al. 1998, 1999; Jho and Carrau 1997; Jho et al. 1996; Resch 1999, 2002; Resch and Perneczky 1994).

■ Dissociation of multiple coordination systems (patient, surgeon, monitors, instruments) (see chap. 5, Fig. 5.9)
The only safe navigation technique is one that can be applied intuitively. Every technical system now brings additional coordination systems into the operative field, which handicaps surgeons as they have to deal with the resulting chaos of incoherent, unsynchronized, and nonconverging coordinates. Surgeons should not be forced to be artists of imaging coordination, but should rather be artists of surgical manipulation.

History of Transendoscopic Sonography

History can guide us to the future, but only if we respect such warnings as the one given by Dagi (1997) about the kind of neurosurgical history currently presented: "The obligation was to a neurosurgical ideal rather than to any individual patient; to an incompletely articulated vision of personal virtue rather than to the profession specifically; and to expression through professional activity rather than through philosophical reflection.". A collection of anecdotes about heroes or a genealogy of the surgeons who did something for the first time will not be very beneficial.

From a neurobiological point of view, history involves documentation and remembering, both of these being essential components of consciousness. Moreover, history can be seen as 'archeology of the brain' and 'phylogenesis of mind' (Resch 1999).

The following short summary of past events is not intended to be a data collection, but rather to give a comprehensive update of the current status, and it focuses on the power of conceptual thinking to create the future.

Endoscopy

Table 1.1 displays a summary – still incomplete – of some specific characteristics of the evolution process.

■ Endoscopes were first used as tools to solve specific problems in hydrocephalus.

Table 1.1. History of endoscopy

1910	Lespinasse	Hydrocephalus	Urethroscope
1918	Dandy	Hydrocephalus	Cystoscope
1919	Payr	Hydrocephalus	Encephaloscopy
1922	Dandy	Obstetric hydrocephalus	Ventriculoscopy, ETV
1923	Volkmann	Hydrocephalus	Encephaloscope
1923	Mixter	Hydrocephalus	ETV with monitor
1923	Fay/Grant	Hydrocephalus	Endoscopic photography
1934	Putnam	Hydrocephalus	Rod lens, diathermy
1936	Scarf	Hydrocephalus	70° lens
1939	Pool	Spinal pathology	Myeloscope
1952	Nulsern/Spitz	Hydrocephalus	Shunt system
1959	Hopkins		Rod-lens endoscope
1963	Guiot	Hydrocephalus colloid cyst Transnasal inspection	Endoscopic light Biportal approach
1973	Fukushima	Hydrocephalus, tumors	Fiberscope, ciné-endoscopy
1974	Prott	CPA	Cisternoscopy
1975	Griffith	Hydrocephalus	Hopkins endoscope
1977	Apuzzo	3rd Ventricular lesions	Stereotaxy and CT guidance
1978	Vries	Hydrocephalus	Large series of ETV
1979	Oppel	Cerebellopontine angle	CPA endoscopy
1983	Auer	Intracerebral hemorrhage	5-Channel endoscope
1987	Gaab	Multiple lesions, tumors	Endoscopy set
1987	Mayer/Brock	Spinal disc lesions	Spinal endoscopy set
1989	Manwaring	Complex cystic lesions	Large series of endoscopic shunting
1989	Bauer/Hellwig	Tumors	Stereotactic fiberscopic biopsies
1990	Caemert	Cysts, ventricles	Stereotactically guided lens-scope
1990	Resch	Endoscopic pathological anatomy	Endoscopic postmortem inspection
1990	Perneczky	All CNS lesions	Endoscopically assisted micro-NC
1992	Karakhan	Ventricular + subarachnoid	Fiberscope
1993	Perneczky et al.	First atlas	Endoscopic anatomy for neurosurgery
1993	Cohen	Ventricular lesions	Large series
1996	Resch	ENS	Transendoscopic sono-guided endoscopy
1996	Grotenhuis	Clinical book	Endoscope-assisted craniotomy
1997	Jho	Skull-base lesions	Extended endoscopic pernasal transsphenoidal neurosurgery

■ After 50 years of neuroendoscopy of the ventricular system and cystic lesions, Guiot used endoscopy by the transnasal approach and Prott, via the CPA, but it was still seen as just a tool.
■ After 80 years of neuroendoscopy, Perneczky's group developed a new concept, which was followed by publication of the first anatomical atlas as revealed by neuroendoscopy. In endoscopy-assisted microneurosurgery the endoscope is by no means just a tool, but has become the cornerstone of a new concept (Perneczky et al. 1993; Resch 1999). This new vision has opened up a wide variety of indications.

■ Finally, Jho took over the ENT concept of endoscopy for pernasal skull-base surgery, in which the microscope is substituted by the endoscope (Cappabianca 1998, 1999; Jho and Carrau 1997; Jho et al. 1996; Resch 1999, 2002). This concept not only enhanced the technical development itself, but also expanded the indications. Interestingly, the history of microneurosurgery shows the same characteristic: not the tool but the new concept led to the brake through.

Neurosonography

In 1937, Dussik used high-frequency sound as a means of diagnosis; French followed in 1950 with ultrasonic pulses used to detect cerebral tumors; and Güttner presented the use of ultrasound imaging in the human skull. In 1956 Leksell then detected the displacement of midline structures by 'echo-encephalography,' and Galicich came up with ultrasound B-scanning of the brain in 1965 (Auer and van Velthoven 1990; Grumme 2001; Strowitzki et al. 2000).

The 1960s saw the introduction of intraoperative ultrasound, but it was not widely accepted because of difficulties in image interpretation. In the 1970s sonography started to be used as an intraoperative imaging technique, and special probes for neurosurgery appeared in the 1980s. In the 1990s color Doppler and power mode became available for intraoperative use (Makuuchi et al. 1998).

Neurosonography was first used in pediatric neurosurgery, as it could be used transcranially (Chadduck 1989; Horwitz and Sorensen 1990; Zorzic and Angonesi 1989). In general neurosurgery sonography was used before that, not only as an ancillary technique to assist those performing open microsurgery (Auer et al. 1988; Auer and van Velthoven 1990; Koivukangas et al. 1993; Mayfrank et al. 1994; Reich et al. 1988; Sutcliffe 1991), but also in stereotactic procedures (Kanazawa et al. 1986; Masuzawa et al. 1985; Moringlane and Voges 1995; Slovis et al. 1991; Tsutsumi et al. 1989; Yamakawa et al. 1994). In 1990 Auer and Velthoven presented their *Atlas of Intraoperative Ultrasound in Neurosurgery*.

The clinical benefit of intraoperative ultrasound has become widely known from works published by several authors (Auer and Velthoven 1990; Suhm et al. 1998; Sutcliffe 1991).

Transendoscopic Sonography

In the 1990s different disciplines started to use the technique of transendoscopic sonography: cardiology (Coy et al. 1991; Müller et al. 1996; Pandian et al. 1993; Roelandt et al. 1993, 1994; Rosenfield et al. 1991; Schwartz et al. 1994), angiology (Aschermann and Fergusson 1992; Aschermann et al. 1992; Cavaye et al. 1991; Delcker and Diener 1994; Isner et al. 1990; Ludwig et al. 1995; Neville et al. 1989), gastroenterology, and urology (Frank et al. 1994; Köstering 1991; Wickham 1993).

One interdisciplinary group, working at the same time as we ourselves were investigating the use of ultrasonography and introducing it in our neurosurgery department, started to use the probe directly, in combination with stereotactic biopsy, in two patients (Froelich et al. 1996). Another group working in pediatric neurosurgery also started to implement it in their clinical practice; both groups, however, failed to achieve informative imaging. In endoscopy it was already a given concept that anatomy should be ahead of surgery, so that starting with anatomical investigations to learn the typical features of the mini-sono-probe and their correlation with endoscopic anatomy was quite normal practice (Grunert et al. 1995; Perneczky et al. 1993; Resch and Perneczky 1993; Resch et al. 1994).

In 1996 we examined the anatomical imaging achieved with endoneurosonography (Resch et al. 1996) as seen in the representation of the ventricular system (Resch and Reisch 1997) and the imaging of the basal cisterns (Resch and Perneczky 1997) with 3D imaging (Resch and Perneczky 1997). In a preliminary series, after our first experience of using the technique in clinical practice, anatomical representation of the spinal chord was included (Resch et al. 1997; Resch and Perneczky 1998).

In March 2002, the first international course on ENS took place in combination with the head-mounted display (HMD) system (www.ens-surgery.com).

Technique and Equipment

Equipment. (Figs. 1.3–1.5) Two different sonocatheters (Aloka and B&K Medical) 1.9 mm (6 F) in diameter have been used; these are introduced into the working channel of an endoscope. The specifications (Aloka/B&K Medical) are:

- Frequency 10, 20 / 12.5 MHz
- Diameter 6 F / 6.2 F
- Length of probe cable 192 / 110 cm
- Display magnification 9–124 mm range in 24 steps
- Frame rate (max.) 15/s
- Image adjustments include gain, STC, contrast, and received frequency bandwidth
- Image rotation through 360°
- Measurement function distance with unit of 0.1 mm
- Display of gray scales, 256 levels
- Video signals TV standard video out and in (BNC)/S-VHS (Y/C)

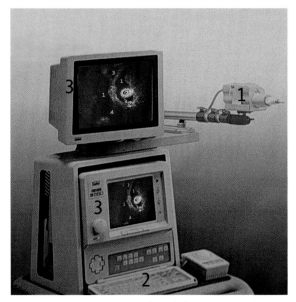

Fig. 1.3. Sono-system. A small mobile conventional sono-graph machine with an additional arm containing the rotation motor for the sono-catheter (*1*). The connector is in contact with the input signal. The keyboard can be used for data input with a variety of imaging parameter configurations (*2*). The image is displayed on two monitors (*3*). Today highend machines are equipped with the technique (Aloka 5000)

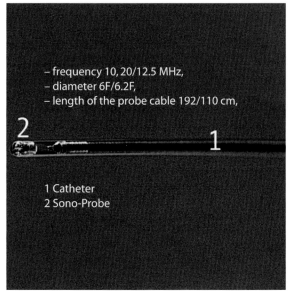

– frequency 10, 20/12.5 MHz,
– diameter 6F/6.2F,
– length of the probe cable 192/110 cm,

1 Catheter
2 Sono-Probe

Fig. 1.4. Sono-probe. The sono-catheter (*1*) has a diameter of 6 F and can be introduced into the working channel of conventional neuroendoscopes. At the tip of the catheter is a mini-sono-probe (*2*). The catheter is inserted in a sterile plastic sheath that has been filled with aqua (not saline). The thin catheter is the only part that appears in the operative field, so that it does not disturb the ergonomics of the working conditions. Another 8-F catheter is used as a sono-dissector outside the endoscope

The Aloka catheter is an elastic cable with a mini-sono-probe at its tip (Fig. 1.4). This catheter is introduced into a sterile plastic sheath. Before the catheter is introduced the sheath is filled with injectable water by means of a thin plastic trocar with a tiny lumen. While the sheath is being filled with liquid (not saline solution) the trocar is carefully withdrawn from the sheath. The sono-catheter is then slowly pushed into the sheath, and care must be taken to ensure that there are no air bubbles in front of the sono-probe at the tip. The tip of the probe is smooth, and there is a 1-mm space between it and the end of the sheath. At this point the prepared sono catheter can be connected with the rotation motor and the signal line. The B&K catheter has a chamber around the mini-sono-probe at its tip, which can be filled with liquid (water) by injection.

The mechanical probes that have been used (ALOKA and B&K) are of type B (Fig. 1.5b). The image provided by use of the probe is a 360° scan ('brain radar') displayed on a monitor, on which some parameters can be varied to get the best view of different anatomical structures.

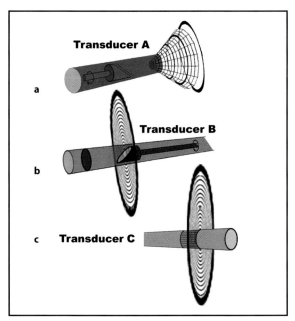

Fig. 1.5a–c. There are two main types of probes, mechanical (a, b) and electronic (c). The ALOKA system is a mechanical type (b), and the probe is rotated by a motor device. (see also Fig. 1.3 (*1*)

Electronic probes are used mainly in cardiology, being designed specifically for near-field investigation with a low penetration depth of a few millimeters. The sono-crystal does not rotate but is configured as a cylindrical array. The low penetration depth is not adequate for use in endo-neuro-sonography.

Imaging Geometry. Scanning geometry (Fig. 1.6a,b: longitudinal, transverse/axial) is important. The representation of a volume scan must be anticipated mentally according to the geometry of scanning. It must be expected that the result of scanning will be represented in a way that is influenced by the geometry of the volume.

The concept of projection geometry is illustrated in Fig. 1.6c: the projection of the scan can be orthogonal to the axial, sagittal, or frontal plane of the anatomy, as it commonly is in CT or MR (Fig. 1.7a,b). Often an oblique projection plane oriented to the pathway of the endoscope in the cranium is used. This is one of the main reasons for difficulties in interpretation of the anatomy visualized by the scan.

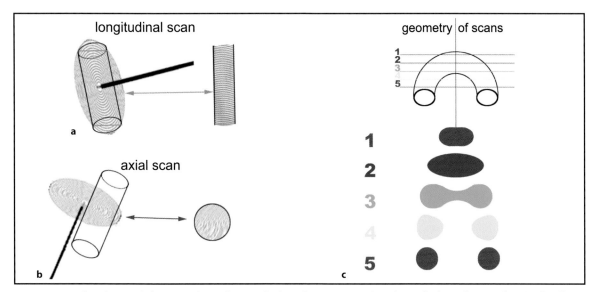

Fig. 1.6. a–c. The shape of the scan depends on whether the scan is going through the volume a longitudinally or b transversely, and also c on the point at which the scan passes through the volume

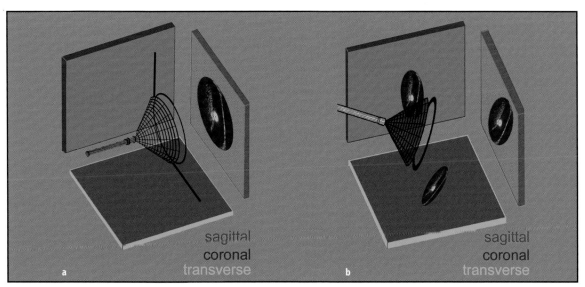

Fig. 1.7a,b. The torsion of the scan in relation to conventional MR or CT planes depends on the angle of the catheter (endoscope) to the orthogonal planes. a When the catheter (endoscope) is parallel to the orthogonal planes a purely axial, sagittal, or frontal scan results. b An angled position of the catheter (endoscope) results in torsion of the scan images

1

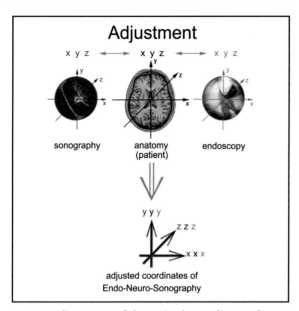

Fig. 1.8. Adjustments of the patient's coordinates, the endoscopic image, and the sonographic image are absolutely essential if ENS is to be a reliable tool for navigation and targeting

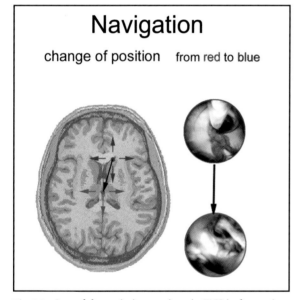

Fig. 1.9. One of the main innovations in ENS is the navigation capacity. The sono-scan at the tip of the endoscope serves as a roadmap of the area around the endoscope. The tip of the endoscope can be seen in this real-time roadmap and is navigated according to the sono-imaging

Adjustment Ability. Just as the color, focus, and orientation of an endoscopic image have to be adjusted, a sonographic image also needs fine-tuning if it is to be useful. It is most important that adjustment of image orientation be done while the focus is on a well-known typical structure with a strong echo signal. Then the orientation focus must be tested by movements of the scope, which in turn must correspond to changes seen on the display of the sonograph. Actual changes of direction and velocity and those seen on the endoscope monitor and the sonograph display must be exactly the same. If this is not the case, the sono-image cannot be correlated with the endoscopic view or interpreted, and competent navigation cannot be achieved (Fig. 1.8).

Navigation Ability (Imaging + Targeting). Endoscopic viewing, even with a limited range and without anatomical mapping outside of this view, appears questionable. In combination with mapping given by the sono-scan ('mini-CT') at the tip of the endoscope, and real-time imaging with the sono-probe, however, endoscopic movements can be mapped in the sono-scan. The tip of the endoscope can be seen as a moving spot on the sono-scan when the endoscope is moved. A target outside the endoscopic view can be reached with online control by sono-scan mapping. This real-time feedback by the sono-scan, representing the starting point and target, fulfills the requirements of navigation. It makes endoscopy intuitively safer (Fig. 1.9).

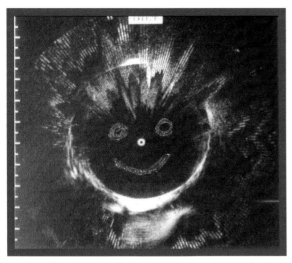

Fig. 1.10. "Artifact-Boy"

3D Sonography

For 3D reconstructions, a postprocessing computer (Tomtec, Munich, Germany) was used to test imaging and handling. For this purpose, the sono-catheter must be driven by hand or, better, automatically in an axial direction while online scanning takes place. The slices are reconstructed on a 3D cylinder of tissue signals. This cylinder can virtually be cut in all three dimensions and displayed with a given rotation movement of a selected angle. This will give a 3D impression of the selected area (Fig. 1.10).

Artifacts

Some effects caused by the equipment itself can lead to a wrong interpretation or distort the image on the screen. Such artifacts can occasionally also be useful for orientation and adjustment. Some of these artifacts seen in ENS are well known in sonography in general, while others are specific to ENS, as illustrated in Figs. 1.11–1.18.

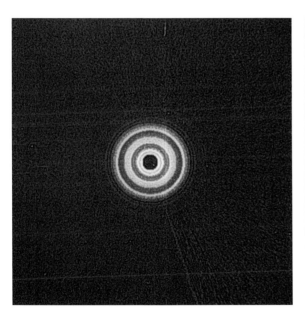

Fig. 1.11. Starting image. Once the sonography machine is started an image of the sono-probe will appear on the display. If this picture does not appear the cause must be investigated and found

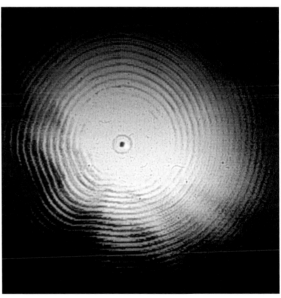

Fig. 1.12. Air artifact. The ENS catheter will typically show an image of this kind if it is not in contact with tissue. This artifact is due to the lack of a contact medium between the crystal and the tissue, which means no imaging will be possible. Occasionally this artifact may detect an air bubble within the CSF, which can be misdiagnosed by the endoscope. The sono-imaging will only work within a fluid medium, so that a clean working field and continuous irrigation are necessary

1

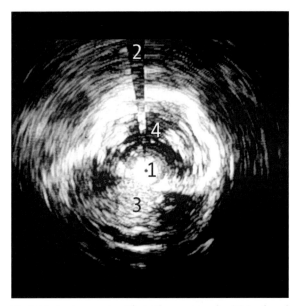

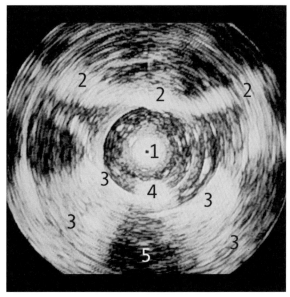

Fig. 1.13. Instrument artifact. The sono-probe (*1*) is placed transnasally in contact with the sella, showing the pituitary gland (*3*). An aspirator placed in the sphenoid sinus (*4*) appears as a typical artifact (*2*). This artifact can easily be recognized as such by moving the instrument

Fig. 1.14. Spatula and cotton artifact. The sono-probe (*1*) is placed by a supraorbital approach along the sphenoid plane (*2*), presenting a frontal scan. The two spatulas placed subfrontally (*3*) are easily recognizable, but a cotton patty (*4*) placed between them to protect the frontal lobe (*5*) could easily be misinterpreted. However, such artifacts are helpful in adjustment of orientation between endoscopic image and sono-image

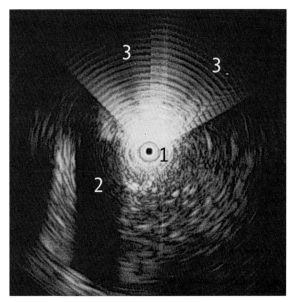

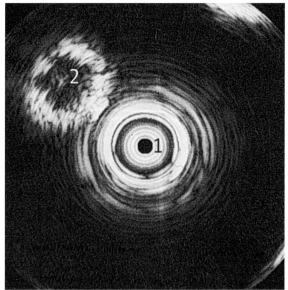

Fig. 1.15. Air bubble artifact. The sono-probe (*1*) is placed in the right frontal horn (*2*). A sectoral air artifact (*3*) is the typical manifestation of an air bubble, which can be misinterpreted on endoscopy because of a mirror effect. The air bubble will look like a mass of tissue in the endoscope, but will be detected at once from the sonographic artifact of air

Fig. 1.16. Lens artifact. If the scanning plane of the sono-probe (*1*) is exactly at the tip of the endoscope an echo-hyperdense ring (*2*) can be seen, which could be misinterpreted as an artery by anyone not familiar with this type of situation

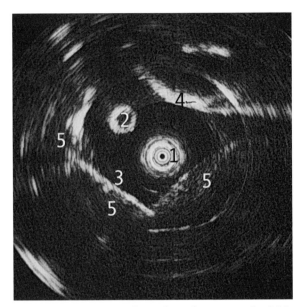

Fig. 1.17. Lens-and-spatula artifact. The sono-probe (*1*) is introduced by a right-sided subtemporal approach, presenting a sagittal scan. The lens artifact (*2*) is visible, in addition to a spatula artifact (*3*). The spatula is lifting the temporal lobe (*5*) from the petrosal bone (*4*)

There are typical artifacts that must be known in the application process. Some of these may impair the imaging, such as an air artifact, while some, such as lens artifacts, can easily be misinterpreted. Some artifacts can be helpful in orientation and targeting, however, and also in the adjustment of image orientation.

Imaging Problems

Sharp bends in the catheter make the scanning uneven, as the cable can stick at some point on its range of rotation (rotation artifact). If the starting image does not appear the cable might not be connected properly. The most frequent reason for missing imaging is the presence of air bubbles in the water around the sono-probe (Fig. 1.15). A problem that is easily overlooked is the lack of any image at all, which arises when isotonic saline solution has been used to fill the sterile sheath.

It must be borne in mind that there might be a defect in the transducer itself, which of course is the worst-case scenario.

The liquid in a cavity, such as a ventricle or the subarachnoid space, should not be too heavily blood stained. Continuous rinsing of the endoscope is the best method of obtaining a clear view in endoscopy and sonography. However, all particles in the CSF, such as protein or blood, will be visible on the sono-scan, which will give an indication of the velocity of CSF flow or irrigation flow.

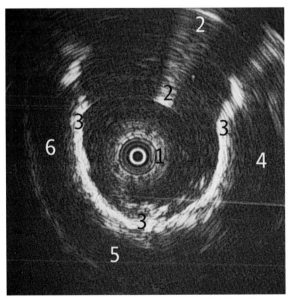

Fig. 1.18. Instrument artifact and burr hole. The sono-probe (*1*) is placed in a burr hole (*3*) at the superior lateral corner in a right lateral-suboccipital approach. The burr hole is sited at the asterion (Janetta approach), where the transverse sinus (*4*) enters the sinus knee (where the sinus makes a 90° bend) (*5*) to become the sigmoid sinus (*6*). An instrument is placed close to the sono-probe (*1*), appearing as a typical instrumental artifact (*2*) on the sono-scan. A scan representing volume must be anticipated in mind with reference to the geometry of the volume

Safety

To date no confirmed harmful biological effects have been identified at the ultrasonic intensity levels recommended for diagnostic use (AIUM 1993; DEGUM 2001; Docker and Duck 1991; EFSUMB 2003; Fowlkes and Holland 2000; Jenne 2001; Koch 2001). In this series, no side effects were identified. The main safety standards are related to the use of electrical equipment.

For actual results see:
- www.aium.org
- www.efsumb.org
- www.ssk.de

Anatomy

Contents

Laboratory Work

The following sonographic anatomical aspects of ENS were established on 21 specimens. After the first clinical series (see chap. 3), the anatomical images were shown from the viewpoint of clinical relevance and only the most typical and relevant examples are reviewed here, with particular attention to principles of imaging (Figs. 2.1, 2.2).

The examinations were done on fresh specimens by different neurosurgical approaches and burr holes. The nonfixed specimens offered the best model in terms of surgery and sono-echo characteristics of tissue.

Work on nonfixed specimens is surprisingly similar to actual surgery, but cannot be planned. This handicap can be compensated by freezing the specimen, which will lead to conditions close to those in fresh preparations when specimens have been thawed for a planned preparation.

Prints, photographs, and parallel sono- and endoscopy video recordings were used for documentation. Modern equipment can also be used to provide digital documentation ready for multimedia use.

The program for presenting ENS involves:
- Different approaches
- Subarachnoid spaces and cisterns
- Important neural and vascular structures
- Endo–sono correlation

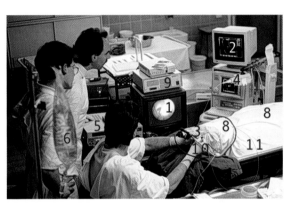

Fig. 2.1. Laboratory setting. Viewing is directed to the endoscopic (*1*) and sonographic (*2*) images, while the endoscope (*3*) is guided freehand. The ENS catheter is connected with the sono-machine (*4*), and only the sono-cable (*11*) comes into the field of vision. A video chain with recorder (*5*), camera machine (*9*) and camera on the endoscope (*3*) is at hand for documentation. The endoscope is equipped with irrigation (*6*), light source (*10*), sono-catheter (*11*) and video chain (*1, 3, 9*). All instruments and endoscopic accessories (*7*) are nearby; the specimen is not fixed, but carefully covered by a sheath (*8*). The laboratory setting is suboptimal. For operative setting see the considerations on ergonomics in Chaps. 1 and 5

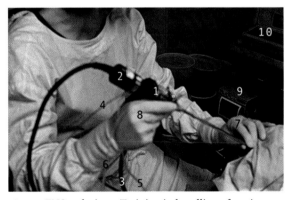

Fig. 2.2. ENS technique. Training in handling of equipment and proficiency testing can be carried out in the laboratory setting. The endoscope (*1*) is equipped with the camera (*2*), the light cable (*3*), irrigation (*4*), suction (*5*) and the sono-catheter (*6*). The endoscope is used freehand but secured at the burr hole with one hand (*7*) and guided with the other (*8*). If one person is working alone, all keyboards (*10*), printers (*9*), etc. must be close and easy to reach with one hand

Questions arising:

- What are the imaging qualities like and what do the anatomical structures look like in sonographic imaging?
- Can the information provided by endoscopy and by endosonography be intuitively correlated?

Effect of Imaging Characteristics on Anatomical Representation

Endoneurosonography adds an axial view of the probe tip's position to the forward view of the endoscope, which itself is visible in the scope and on the sonographic view. This axial vision is like an axial 'mini-CT' of the tip plane on which the position of the tip itself can be localized in relation to the axial anatomy. The zoom function makes it possible to adapt the view in relation to the size of structures. It is possible to see an overall picture of some 6 cm or to see only one small cistern of some millimeters in diameter. In addition, it allows anticipation of the aspects that will come into view in the endoscope next, by 'looking through the parenchyma' and viewing a larger overall area than the scope does. The 'online mode' of the sono-view allows changes of structures, such as changing size of ventricles and shifting of the parenchyma, to be observed, as well as pulsation or blood flow in the vessels. When used in combination with the endo-view, it allows safe neuronavigation of the scope online and in real time.

For such problems as intraoperative imaging or navigation of the endoscope, the imaging characteristic (Figs. 2.3, 2.4) for structures 4 cm or less in diameter is comparable to that of CT. A small cyst of the pellucid septum was visible in the sono, for example, as well as retrospectively in the CT. There are, however, important differences between CT imaging and endo-sono imaging:

- The geometry of the sono-scan shows torsion representing the angle of the scope, as well as the angle of the catheter to the plane of the CT scan in the sagittal and coronary planes.
- The sono-scan shows the CSF/tissue border and the choroid plexus more strongly than they appear in the CT scan.
- The sono-scan gives an online and real-time image, in contrast to intraoperative CT.
- The sono-scan shows movements, such as a change in ventricle shape or blood flow in the vessels, representing physiological parameters.

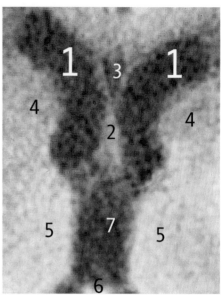

Fig. 2.3. Cavum of pellucid septum/CT. The CT scan shows a clasp of the midline structures. Frontal horns of lateral ventricles (*1*) are divided by the pellucid septum (*2*), which presents a small cyst (*3*). The septum ends at the fornices, where both foramina of Monro enter the third ventricle. The frontal horns are bordering the caudate nuclei (*4*) laterally and the third ventricle, formed by the thalamus (*5*), on both sides. The hyperdense pineal body (*6*) is clearly visible, marking the dorsal end of the third ventricle (*7*)

Fig. 2.4. Cavum of septum scan. The sono-scan is concentrated in this close-up of the frontal horns (1) with pellucid septum (2) between, clearly representing the cyst (3) that was visible on CT. Both foramina of Monro (4) are visible, plus the choroid plexus (5), which appears at higher echodensity than in the CT. The CSF/tissue border is also represented much more strongly on the sono-scan than on the CT scan. The sono-scan shows the typical torsion of geometry according to the angle of the endoscope plus catheter to the CT plane in the sagittal and coronal dimensions. The sono-probe (6) is visible in the right frontal horn, while the tip of the endoscope in the sono-probe is presented in the anatomy precisely and in real time. Movements and direction of movements of the scope are visible online and in real time

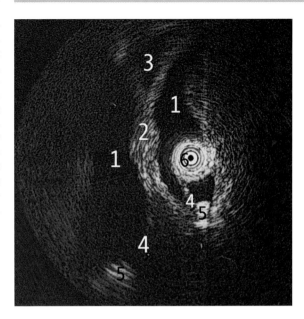

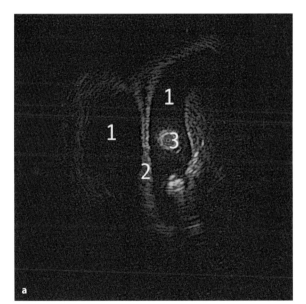

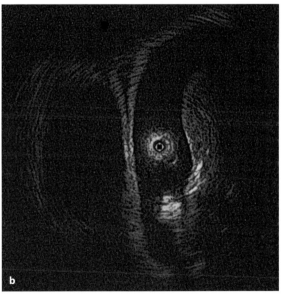

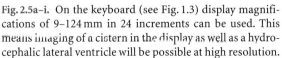

Fig. 2.5a–i. On the keyboard (see Fig. 1.3) display magnifications of 9–124 mm in 24 increments can be used. This means imaging of a cistern in the display as well as a hydrocephalic lateral ventricle will be possible at high resolution.

Both frontal horn (1) and septum (2) are zoomed until only structures within 9 mm of the sono-probe (3) are visible without loss of optical resolution, but the noise artifact will become more intense

2

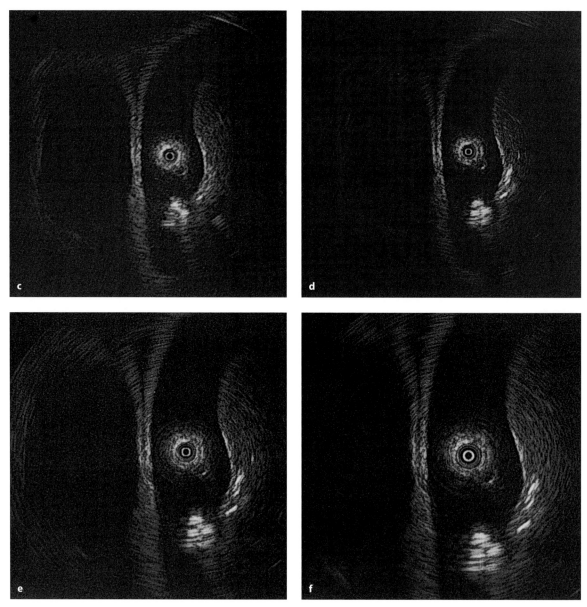

Fig. 2.5c–f.

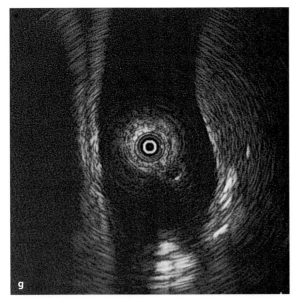

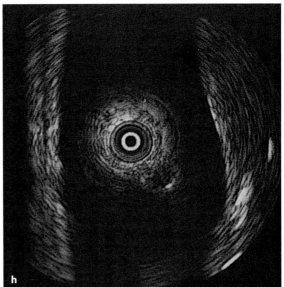

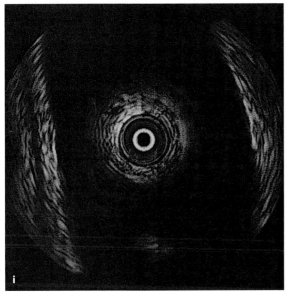

Fig. 2.5g–i.

2

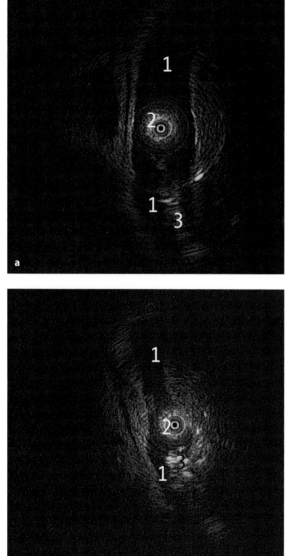

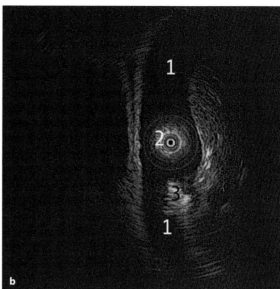

Fig. 2.6a–c. The ENS catheter detects and displays volume changes. The ventricular volume (*1*) is shown becoming progressively smaller from a to c as a result of CSF evacuation. Eventually the ventricular walls and the choroid plexus (*2*) come close to the sono-probe (*3*)

Zoom Effect and Change of Volume

The zoom effect and change in volume are seen particularly well in the cases illustrated in Figs. 2.5 and 2.6.

This gives possibility to adapt the scan to the anatomy and to the needs of imaging.

Illustrative Anatomical Cases

The sono-scan shows the well-known anatomy and endoscopic anatomy in very typical slices and shapes with a high significance in recognition and easy correlation to the optical visualization. Once some experience has indicated what can be visualized and what can be expected, intuitive handling and interpretation of the standard images will soon result. Some *typical examples* of imaging are described below:

Ventricular System. During their progression through the ventricular system, the shape of the scan image varies according to the position of the sono-probe and the tip of the endoscope: the endoscope gives the typical 3D view in front of the lens into a given space showing the typical landmarks of the right lateral ventricle.

The sono-scan not only shows the right ventricle, but also visualizes both ventricles in 2D like a CT and also gives a view into the parenchyma. The contact of the sono-probe with the choroid plexus is well controlled by the endoscope and represented exactly in the sono-scan (Figs. 2.7–2.20)

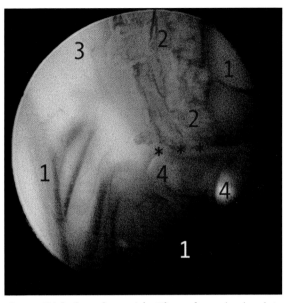

Fig. 2.7. Right lateral ventricle. The endoscopic view into the right lateral ventricle (*1*) shows the choroid plexus (*2*) and the pellucid septum (*3*) at the level of the sella media. The sono-probe (*4*) is optically controlled while in contact (***) with the plexus (*2*)

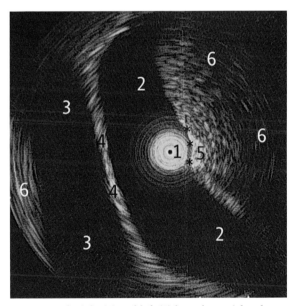

Fig. 2.8. Both right (*2*) and left (*3*) lateral ventricles shown by sono-scan. The probe (*1*) itself is visible at the *right*, in contact (***) with the choroid plexus (*5*). Moreover it can 'see' through the pellucid septum (*4*) and into the parenchyma (*6*)

2

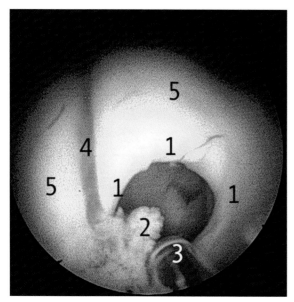

Fig. 2.9. Foramen of Monro. The endoscope is in front of the right foramen of Monro, which is formed by the fornix (1) and the choroid plexus (2). The sono-probe (3) is controlled optically by the endoscope and pushed a little way into the foramen. A septum vein (4) crosses over the pellucid septum (5)

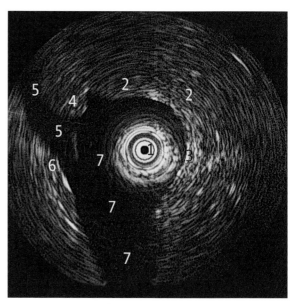

Fig. 2.10. Foramen of Monro. The sono-probe (1) is just in the right foramen of Monro formed by the fornix (2) and choroid plexus (3). In contrast to the endoscope, the sonoscan represents the left fornix in an axial cut (4) and also the left foramen of Monro (5). The left choroid plexus too is just in the scan (6), and the whole length of the third ventricle (7) is displayed

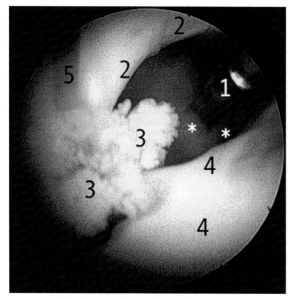

Fig. 2.11. Third ventricle. Under endoscopic control, the sono-probe (1) is pushed into the third ventricle towards the mamillary bodies (*). The fornix (2), the choroid plexus (3), and the anterior part of the thalamus covered by lamina affixa (4) form the foramen of Monro. The septum vein (5) crosses the fornix (2)

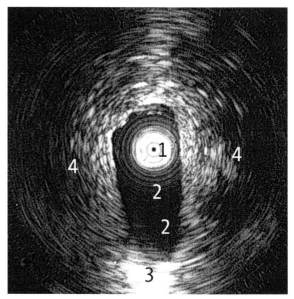

Fig. 2.12. Third ventricle scan. The sono-probe (1) is in the third ventricle (2), limited by the thalamus (4) on both sides and by the pineal body (3)

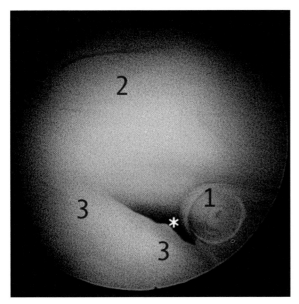

Fig. 2.13. Aqueduct. The sono-probe (*1*) is entering the aqueduct (*) at the posterior third ventricle formed by hypothalamus (*2*) and posterior commissure (*3*)

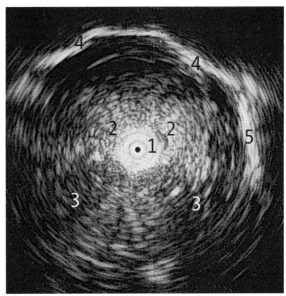

Fig. 2.14. Aqueduct and posterior fossa. The sono-probe (*1*) is inside the aqueduct of the mesencephalon (*2*). As the zoom is very low, the posterior fossa is scanned with the cerebellum (*3*), clivus, and petroclival border (*4*), plus the tentorial notch on the right side (*5*)

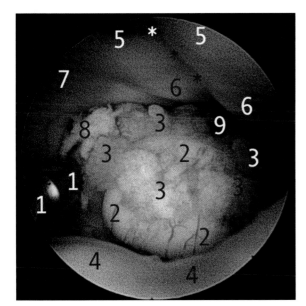

Fig. 2.15. Fourth ventricle. The sono-probe (*1*) is inside the fourth ventricle under visual control. The inferior vermis (*2*) is bulging into the ventricle covered by the variant of a circular plexus (*3*). The superior medullary velum (*4*) limits the inferior view while a view into the depth of the foramen of Magendi (*9*) is possible. The surface of the rhombencephalon shows the facial colliculus (*6*) and medial eminence (*5*) on both sides, divided by the medial sulcus (*). Laterally, the vestibular area (*7*) is visible, as is the entry to the foramen of Luschka (*8*)

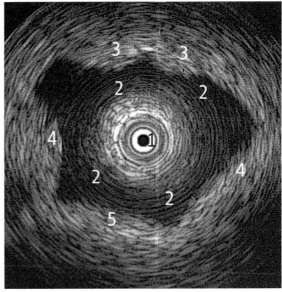

Fig. 2.16. Fourth ventricle scan. The sono-probe (*1*) is in the fourth ventricle looking into the parenchyma of facial colliculus (*3*), superior cerebellar peduncle (*4*), and superior medullary velum and superior vermis (*5*)

2

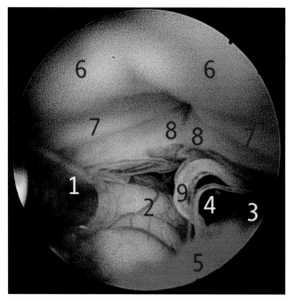

Fig. 2.17. Inferior fourth ventricle. The endoscope enters the ventricle, controlling the sono-probe (*1*) and touching the plexus (*5*). The left (*2*) and right (*3*) cerebellar tonsils lead to the foramen of Magendi (*4*), where a circumflex tonsillar artery (*9*) is visible. The typical surface of the rhombencephalon contains facial colliculus (*6*), medullary striae (*7*) and hypoglossal triangle (*8*)

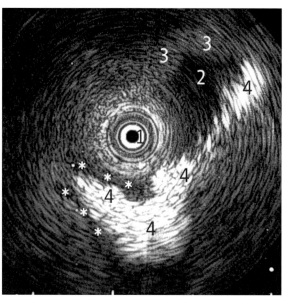

Fig. 2.18. Inferior fourth ventricle scan. The sono-probe (*1*) is now in the lateral fourth ventricle. In the middle of the ventricle (*2*), facial colliculi are visible on both sides (*3*) and the choroid plexus (*4*) can be followed into the lateral recess (*)

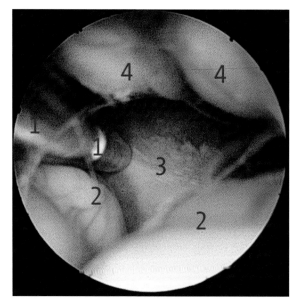

Fig. 2.19. Cisterna magna. The sono-probe (*1*) is guided along the cerebellar tonsils (*2*) into the cisterna magna (*3*) with endoscopic vision. The ventral medulla oblongata (*4*) extends into the foramen magnum

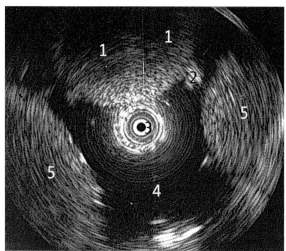

Fig. 2.20. Cisterna magna scan. The sono-probe (*3*) is introduced into the cisterna magna (*4*) close to the medulla (*1*). Laterally, both cerebellar tonsils (*5*) are visible and the right vertebral artery (*2*) is scanned

Ventral Cisterns. Like the ventricles, cisterns are ideal subjects for both endoscopy and endosonography. The 2D anatomical example presented is the interpeduncular cistern. This cistern is the target area in the procedure of endoscopic third ventriculocisternostomy (ETV).

The endoscope is inserted through a precoronal mediopupillary burr hole and advanced transcerebrally into the frontal horn. It is then passed through the foramen of Monro, and the endoscope is placed above the anterior floor of the third ventricle. The endoscopically visible landmarks for penetration are the mamillary bodies, the tuber cinereum, and the infundibular recess. In a translucent membranous cinereum (premamillary membrane) the dorsum of the sella is visible, and at times also the basilar tip. If the floor is bulging the infundibulum is wide open and the stalk is flattened to look like a red spot. The scope should penetrate between the dorsum of the sella and the basilar head.

This route can be navigated by endo-sono instrumentation. Especially in small ventricles, the sono-catheter can be advanced through the parenchyma ahead of the endoscope, which does not see, whilst the sono-probe will 'see' its position as it enters the ventricle. The endoscope can then use the sono-catheter as a guidewire. Once both instruments have entered the frontal horn, both images, endoscopic and sonographic, are visible. The endoscope will look ahead into the infundibulum and onto the floor of the third ventricle, while the sono-probe will 'see' the thalamus and then the hypothalamus, and also the vessels of the circle of Willis and what blood flow there is.

If the floor is not translucent the sono-probe can be advanced as a 'seeing' catheter and will show the position of the basilar artery, the posterior communicating arteries, both oculomotor nerves, and of course the dorsum of the sella before the endoscope is advanced (Figs. 2.21–2.35).

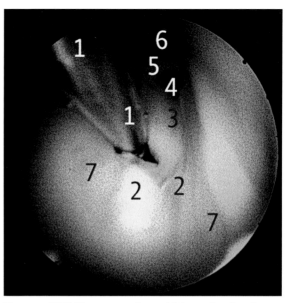

Fig. 2.21. ETV. The sono-catheter (*1*) is perforating the tuber cinereum (*3*) anterior to the mamillary bodies (*2*). The endoscopic view does not see now the anatomy of interpeduncular cistern. The further topographical points are the infundibular recess (*4*), the optic chiasm (*5*), the supraoptic recess (*6*), and the walls of the hypothalamus (*7*)

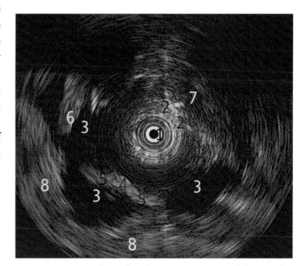

Fig. 2.22. Interpeduncular cistern. In a near axial scan, the sono-probe (*1*) shows the basilar artery (*4*) as a hyperdense spot, both P1 segments (*5*) spreading laterally on both sides, and the dorsum of sella (*2*) as a strong hyperdense line. These are the main landmarks, which the sono probe may already 'see' even before penetrating the floor of the third ventricle. When placed in the interpeduncular cistern (*3*) it can image the oculomotor nerve (*6*) and the brain stem (*8*) and the view into the parenchyma of the pituitary gland (*7*)

2

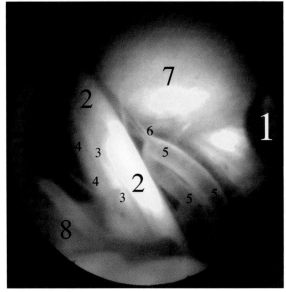

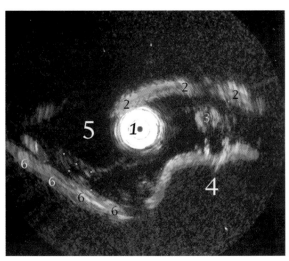

Fig. 2.23. Cerebellopontine angle (CPA). The endoscopic view from superior direction into the left CPA depicts the sono-probe (*1*), inferior to the 7/8 boundle with a facial nerve (*2*), intermedial nerve (*3*), and the acoustic nerve (*4*). An ICA loop (*5*) with a branching labyrinthine artery (*6*) is clearly visualized. The probe (*1*) is in contact with the petrous bone (*7*)

Fig. 2.24. CPA scan. The sono-probe (*1*) is in contact with the lateral clivus (*2*) positioned in the left CPA (*5*) with the 7/8 boundle (*6*) and the ICA loop (...). Moreover the pons (*4*) and basilar artery (*3*) are visible

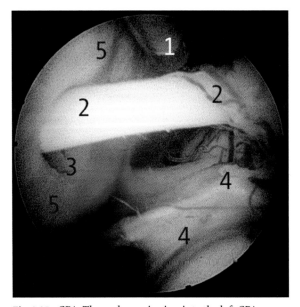

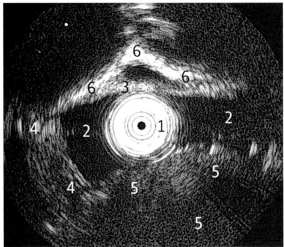

Fig. 2.25. CPA. The endoscopic view into the left CPA represents the sono-probe (*1*) inferior to the 7/8 boundle (*2*), running into the acoustic meatus (*3*) and medial to the petrous bone (*5*). The inferior lateral part of the pons (*4*) is bulging out in this unusual view from above

Fig. 2.26. CPA scan. The sono-probe (*1*) is in the left CPA cistern (*2*) in contact with the pons (*5*) and an arachnoid membrane (*3*). The 7/8 boundle (*4*) runs towards the petrous bone (*6*)

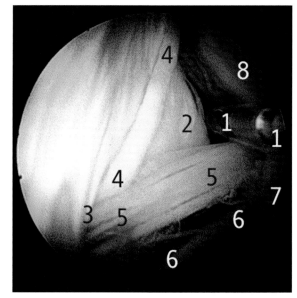

Fig. 2.27. Jugular foramen. The endoscope looks on the jugular foramen (3), while the sono-probe (1) is in contact with the jugular tubercle (2). Accessory nerve (4), vagus fibers (5) and glossopharyngeal nerve (6) enter their dural pores (3). The sono-probe (1) is also in contact with 'Bochdalek's' body (7) and the medulla (8)

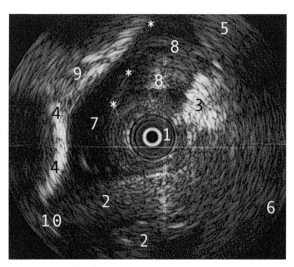

Fig. 2.28. Jugular foramen scan. The sono-probe (1) is positioned in the lateral cerebellomedullary cistern (inferior CPA cistern) (7). In contrast to the endoscopic view (Fig. 2.27), the position is now superior to the vagus fibers (8), running to the jugular foramen (9) and in contact with Bochdalek's body (3), pons (6), and medulla (5). An arachnoid membrane (*) is hardly visible. The 7/8 boundle (2) runs towards the petrous bone (4) to the acoustic meatus (10)

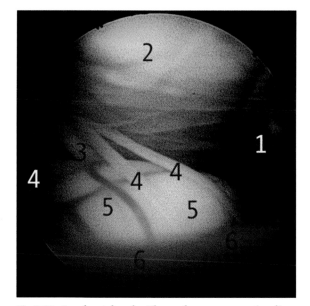

Fig. 2.29. Jugular tubercle. The endoscope now visualizes the sono-probe (1) touching the right jugular tubercle (2). The vertebral artery (6) and fibers of the vagus nerve (4) cross the olive (5) and then run together with the accessory nerve (3) to the jugular foramen

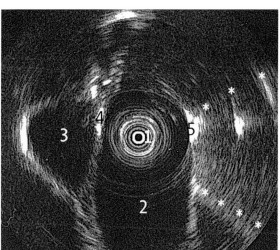

Fig. 2.30. Jugular tubercle scan. The sono-probe (1) is lateral to the cerebellomedullary cistern (2) close to the jugular tubercle (4), visualizing the sigmoid sinus at the jugular bulb level (3) through the thin bony layer of the jugular tubercle (4)

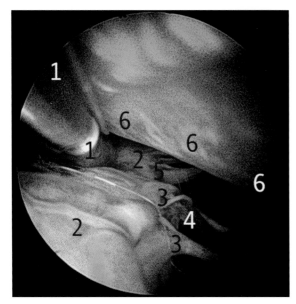

Fig. 2.31. Foramen magnum. The endoscope is looking at the anterior border of the foramen magnum (6). The sono-probe (1) touches the foramen and the medulla (2) at C-1 level. Below this the right C-2 root (5), and above it the C-1 root (3) are accompanied by a laterally medullary vein (4) leaving the medulla

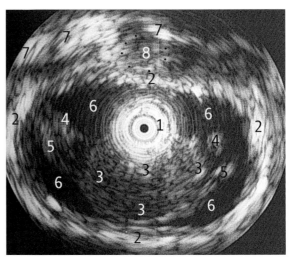

Fig. 2.32. Foramen magnum scan. The sono-probe (1) is placed in the lower foramen magnum, ventral to the medulla spinalis at C-2 level (3). The dural border of the foramen magnum is present (2), as is the ventral bony border (7) where the dens axis is hardly visible (8, ·····). In the spinal subarachnoid space (6) the ventral (4) and dorsal (5) roots are visible on both sides

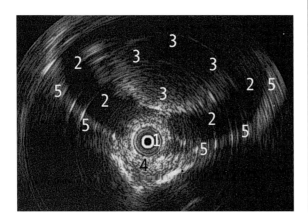

Fig. 2.33. Atlas-level scan. The sono-probe (1) is placed dorsal to the medulla (3) in the spinal subarachnoid space (2), touching the dorsal arch of the atlas (5) at the posterior tubercle (4). The scan is overlaid by the rotation artifact caused by uneven rotation of the ENS cable in the sheath

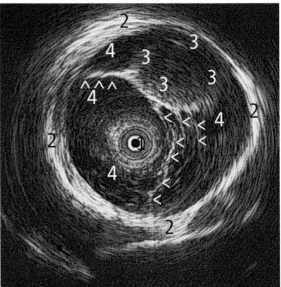

Fig. 2.34. Thoracic spinal canal scan. The sono-probe (1) is placed in the thoracic subarachnoid space (4) dorsal to the medulla (3) close to the dorsal subarachnoid septum (<) with some subarachnoid membranes (<). On the left side a dental ligament (^^^) within the scan is completely surrounded by the dural and bony border (2) of the spinal canal

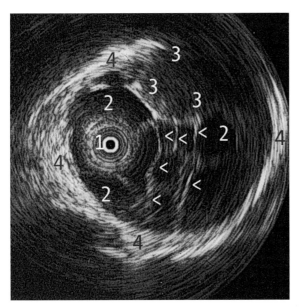

Fig. 2.35. Thoracic spinal canal scan. The sono-probe (*1*) is placed in the thoracic spinal subarachnoid space (*2*) dorsal to the medulla (*3*) and close to a network of arachnoid membranes (<), surrounded by the bony border of the canal (*4*)

Suprasellar and Retrosellar Space. When the subarachnoid space and the cisterns are to be imaged, endoscopy must be accompanied by irrigation, as the sono-probe needs a liquid medium to show up any findings. In the example presented the scope is inserted through a lateral supraorbital burr hole approaching the chiasmatic cistern with both optic nerves. In this case of a wide-open prechiasmatic window, the pituitary stalk and diaphragm of the sella are visible. Depending on the anatomical circumstances the endoscope can sometimes reach the posterior fossa, but in our case only the sono-probe, which was optically controlled, was advanced so far. This means that the sono-probe scans the suprasellar and sellar space in a semi-sagittal manner.

The sono-scan presents the sella with the entire parenchyma of the pituitary gland. Both the stalk and the left optic nerve are visible, and in contrast to the endoscopic view the anterior part of the third ventricle is visualized (Figs. 2.36–2.44).

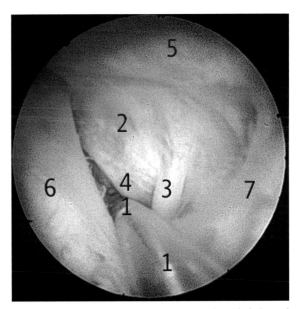

Fig. 2.36. Suprasellar space. From a right-sided lateral supraorbital burr hole, the endoscope approaches the suprasellar space. The chiasmatic cistern is visible, with left (*6*) and right (*7*) optic nerves, pituitary stalk (*3*) and diaphragm of sella (*2*). Under optical control, the sono-probe (*1*) is pushed along the left posterior clinoid process (*4*)

2

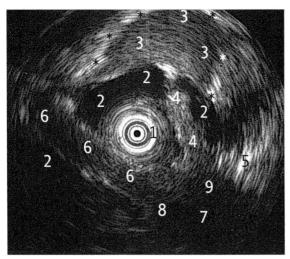

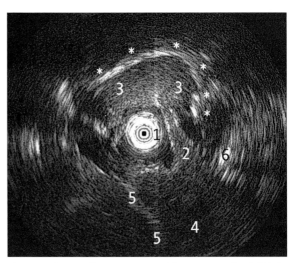

Fig. 2.37. Suprasellar space scan. The sono-scan and the sono-probe (1) are located in the chiasmatic cistern (2), representing a semisagittal imaging plane. The sella (*) with the parenchyma of the pituitary gland (3) and the stalk (4) with the left optic nerve (6) are visible. In contrast to the endoscope, the sono-probe (1) can 'see' into the anterior third ventricle (7) with infundibular (9) and supraoptic recess (8). The dorsum of the sella (5) is visible

Fig. 2.38. Suprasellar space scan. The sono-probe (1) is in the suprasellar space close to the pituitary stalk (2) and the pituitary gland (3) in the sella (*). The anterior third ventricle (4) with lamina terminalis (5) is visible. The basilar artery (6) gives a high signal (6)

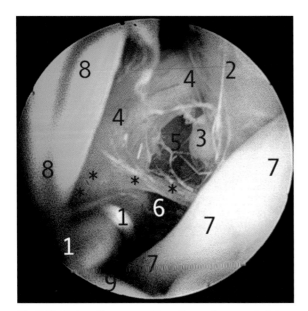

Fig. 2.39. Retrosellar space. Now the endoscope is introduced into the retrosellar space from a right laterosuboccipital approach and the sono-probe (1) is advanced over the right P1 segment (9) and oculomotor nerve (7) under a strong posterior communicating artery (8) into the interpeduncular cistern (6). The anterior arachnoid wall (*) is visible curving into the Lilliequist's membrane and separating this cistern from the peri-infundibular subarachnoid space ('inferior chiasmatic cistern') (5). Dorsum of the sella (2) and the contralateral left posterior clinoid process (3) are visible. The pituitary stalk (4) enters the sella

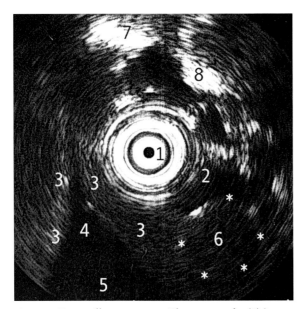

Fig. 2.40. Retrosellar space scan. The sono-probe (*1*) is now placed in the retrosellar space (*2*) close to the infundibulum (*3*). In contrast to the endoscopic view, the scan presents the view into the anterior third ventricle (*5*) with the infundibular recess (*4*). A mamillary body (*6*) is visible with the dorsum of the sella (*7*) and the clivus (*8*)

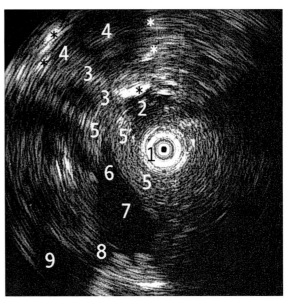

Fig. 2.41. Retrosellar space scan. The sono-probe (*1*) is placed in the retrosellar space (*2*) close to the infundibulum (*5*) and the stalk (*3*), which enters the sella (*) and pituitary gland (*4*). The anterior third ventricle (*7*) is visible, leading into the infundibular recess (*6*) caudally and the foramen of Monro (*8*) cranially, and into a lateral ventricle (*9*)

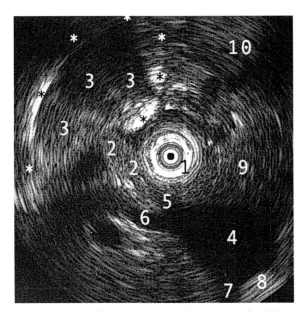

Fig. 2.42. Retrosellar space scan. The sono-probe (*1*) is placed in the interpeduncular cistern close to the infundibulum and stalk (*2*). The sella (*) and pituitary gland (*3*), mesencephalon (*9*), and pons (*10*) are visible. The anterior third ventricle (*4*) with infundibular recess (*5*), supraoptic recess (*6*), and foramen of Monro (*7*) and the choroid plexus (*8*) are present

2

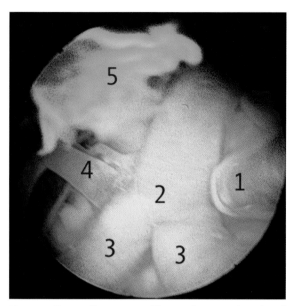

Fig. 2.43. Retrosellar space. The endoscope is placed through a pterional approach into the interpeduncular cistern with the basilar head (*2*), which is touched by the sono-probe (*1*) under visual control with the two branching posterior communicating arteries (*3*) and the left superior cerebellar artery (SuCA) (*4*). The arachnoid membrane (*5*) is floating in the visual field

Ventriculo- and Ventrocisternal ENS – Route in a 1-year-old Child. The endoscopic images recorded in children and premature newborns differ substantially from those in adults. There is as yet no standard work available showing the typical differences and variations. The shapes of the sono-scans shown above also differ from those seen in the next, axial, series and may at first give a casuistic impression about this (Figs. 2.45–2.59).

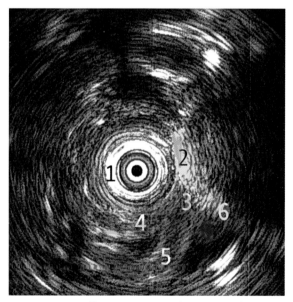

Fig. 2.44. Retrosellar space scan. The sono-probe (*1*) is moved from the pterional into the interpeduncular cistern to the left side of the basilar artery (*2*), which branches into the left SuCA (*4*), left P1 (*5*), and right P1 (*6*). In this way almost all of the basilar head (*3*) is scanned in a frontal plain

Fig. 2.45. MRT. On the axial MR, the route (°) through the ventricular system and the ventral cisterns is marked

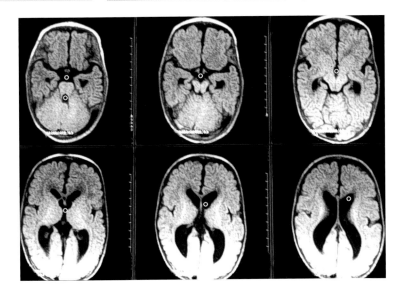

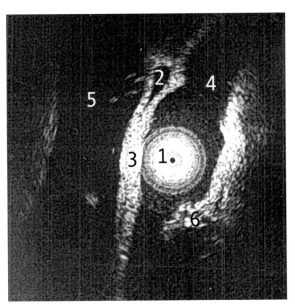

Fig. 2.46. Lateral ventricles. The sono-probe (1) is placed in the right frontal horn touching the pellucid septum (3). The septum cyst (2) seen on the MR (Fig. 2.33), is clearly visible, as are the left frontal horn (5) and the choroid plexus (6)

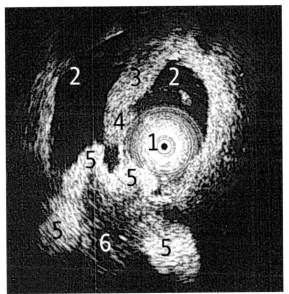

Fig. 2.47. Choroid plexus. The sono-probe (1) is just at the level of the foramina of Monro, where the choroid plexus (5) runs through from the lateral ventricle (2) to the roof of the third ventricle (6). The septum (3) and both fornices (4) separate the frontal horn (2)

2

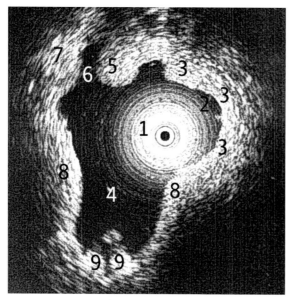

Fig. 2.48. Foramen of Monro level. The sono-probe (*1*) is just in the right foramen of Monro (*2*) formed by the fornix (*3*) and entering the third ventricle (*4*). The contralateral fornix (*5*) and foramen of Monro (*6*) are visualized. Left caput of caudate nucleus (*7*), both thalami (*8*), and the plexus (*9*) at the roof of the third ventricle (*4*) are visible

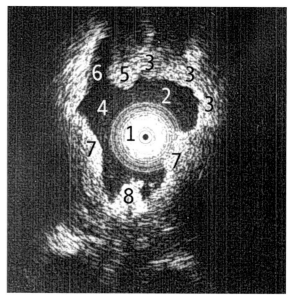

Fig. 2.49. Foramen of Monro level. The sono-probe (*1*) has now been advanced a little further into the third ventricle (*4*), but is still in the foramen of Monro (*2*) formed by the fornix (*3*). Left fornix (*5*) and foramen of Monro (*6*), both anterior thalami (*7*), and choroid plexus (*8*) are seen

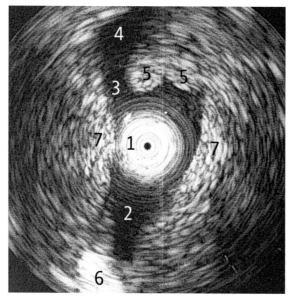

Fig. 2.50. Third ventricle. The sono-probe (*1*) has entered the third ventricle (*2*) and can depict the contralateral left foramen of Monro (*3*) and a small part of the frontal horn (*4*). Both fornices (*5*) and thalami (*7*) are pictured, as is the pineal body (*6*)

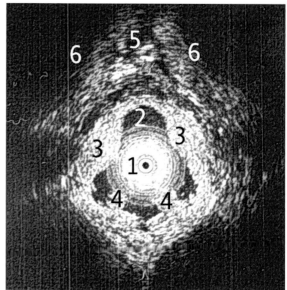

Fig. 2.51. Hypothalamus. The sono-probe (*1*) is located at the beginning of the infundibulum (*2*). The walls of the hypothalamus (*3*) on both sides are visible, while the mamillary bodies (*4*) are just coming into the scan. Outside the ventricle, the frontal lobes (*6*) with the midline and right A2 with communicating anterior artery (CoA) (*5*) are present

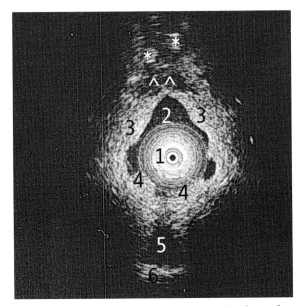

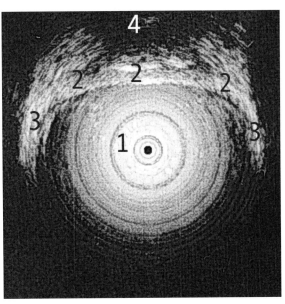

Fig. 2.52. Hypothalamus. The sono-probe (*1*) is located at the entrance of the infundibulum (*2*) formed by the hypothalamus (*3*). The mamillary bodies (*4*) are in contact with the probe (*1*) and posterior to the beginning of the aqueduct (*5*); the posterior commissure (*6*) is visible. Outside the ventricle, the frontal midline with both anterior cerebral arteries (A2; *) and CoA (^^) is noticeable

Fig. 2.53. Sella level. The sono-probe (*1*) is placed at the dorsum of the sella (*2*). Laterally the petroclival ligament is attached (*3*). Through the bone of the clivus (dorsum) (*2*) the sella (*4*) is visible in an axial scan

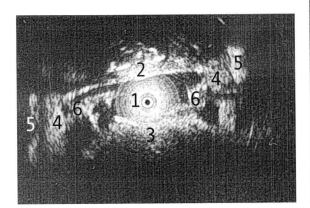

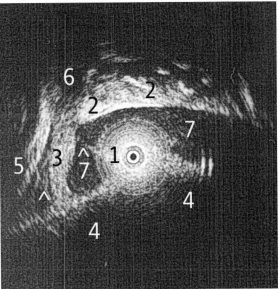

Fig. 2.54. Prepontine cistern level. The sono-probe (*1*) is in touch with the clivus (*2*) and the pons (*3*). On both sides, the trigeminal nerves (*4*) with part of SuCA (*6*) and the tentorium (*5*) are present

Fig. 2.55. Trigeminal nerve (*5*)level. The sono-probe (*1*) is in the prepontine cistern (*7*), touching the pons (*4*) and close to the clivus (*2*). This close-up view shows the trigeminal nerve (*3*) crossing the subarachnoid space (*7*) and entering Meckel's cavity (*6*) with its arachnoid sheath (^)

2

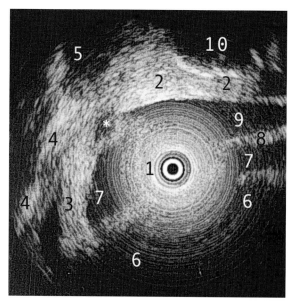

Fig. 2.56. Trigeminal nerve level. The sono-probe (*1*) is located in the prepontine cistern (*7*) covered by the arachnoid membrane (*8*). Outside the membrane (*8*) the epiarachnoid space (*9*) appears. The clivus (*2*) ends laterally at the cavernous sinus (*5*), where the trigeminal nerve (*3*) enters its dural porus (***) beneath the tentorium (*4*). The sono-probe touches the pons (*6*). In the clivus (*2*) a small sphenoid sinus (*10*) becomes visible

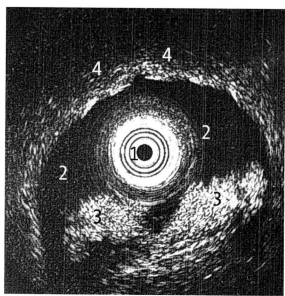

Fig. 2.57. Fourth ventricle. The sono-probe (*1*) is located in the fourth ventricle (*2*). Ventrally the surface of the rhombencephalon with facial colliculus (*4*) is visible, while dorsally the choroid plexus (*3*) is present

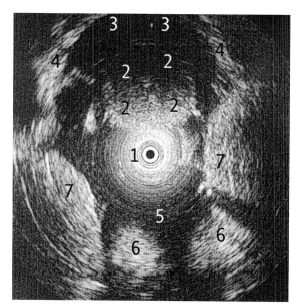

Fig. 2.58. Cisterna magna level. The sono-probe (*1*) is placed at the cisterna magna (*5*) and has made contact with the dorsal surface of the medulla (*2*). Ventral to the medulla (*2*), the premedullary cistern (*3*) and the clivus (*4*) are visible. Dorsally, the tonsils (*6*) and lobus biventer (*7*) are present

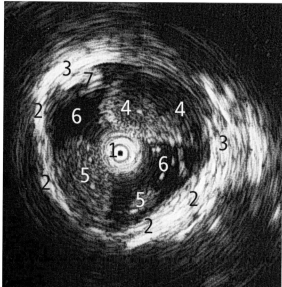

Fig. 2.59. Foramen magnum. The sono-probe (*1*) is placed in the foramen magnum (*2*) and in the subarachnoid space of the cisterna magna (*6*) dorsal to the medulla (*4*) and ventral to the tonsils (*5*). At the bony border of the foramen magnum (*2*), laterally, the occipital condyles (*3*) are visible, as is the vertebral artery on the *left side* (*7*)

3D Anatomy of Midline Structures. The initial re-sults of 3D postprocessing on two adults and a 1-year-old child showed the ventricles and the tissue around the sono-catheter, presenting a cylindrical volume with the penetration depth as the radius and the catheter's course as the length of the cylinder. On the display, this volume moves in the selected manner with reference to rotation, angle, and frequency. The ventricles of a 1-year-old child (Figs. 2.45–2.59) are reconstructed in coronal and sagittal views. For 3D reconstruction it is necessary to move the catheter very steadily.

The 3D volume can be cut in different planes. In the example, a mediosagittal plane is cut and the view into the third ventricle from the lateral direction is shown. The sono-catheter is visible in the reconstruc-tion as it passes through the foramen of Monro, through the floor of the third ventricle, and into the interpeduncular cistern behind the dorsum of the sella. This is, so to speak, a 3D representation of a third ventriculocisternostomy (Figs. 2.60–2.62).

Fig. 2.60. a Axial and b frontal slice reconstruc-tions of a transendoscopic sonography. The *yellow line* in a indicates the position of the frontal plane shown in b. The ENS catheter (*1*) is introduced through the right frontal horn (*2*), passing through the right foramen of Monro (*3*) into the third ventricle (*4*). It then runs through an ETV along the prepontine cistern (*5*) and into the spinal canal (*6*)

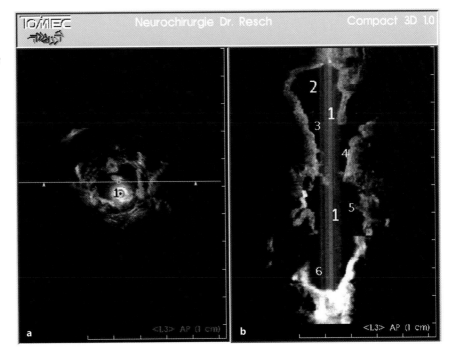

2

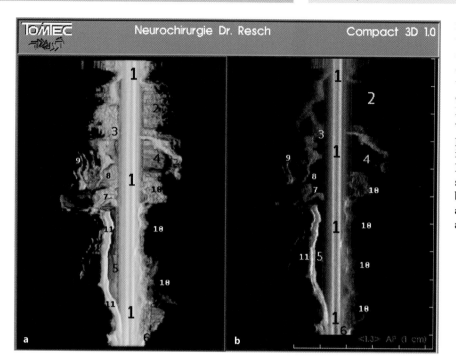

Fig. 2.61. a 3D and b sagittal reconstruction in one slice, showing the passage of the ENS catheter (*1*) through the lateral ventricle (*2*), the foramen of Monro (*3*), and the third ventricle (*4*) along the prepontine cisterns (*5*) into the spinal canal (*6*). Infundibular recess (*7*), supraoptic recess (*8*), both anterior cerebral arteries (*9*), brain stem (*10*) and clivus (*11*) can be seen

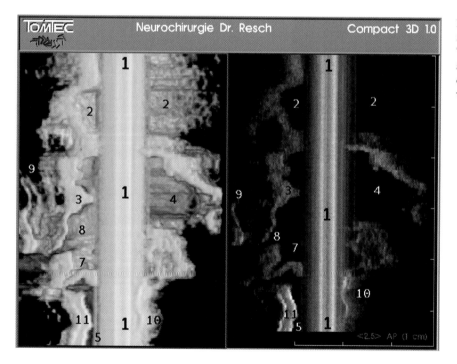

Fig. 2.62. Sagittal reconstruction of third ventricle. This close-up of the slice shown in Fig. 61b shows detail around the third ventricle in a sagittal slice

Transnasal ENS Anatomy of Sellar Region. The transnasal approach is a minimally invasive one, and the small size and deep channel limit the light power of the microscope. Only a part of the light will reach the deepest tissue being viewed, and magnification will result in a dark image with a very short focus depth. It is in these conditions that the endoscope is superior to the microscope, as it travels into the anatomy, placing the optic keyhole closer to the target. This is also the case in sonography by ENS.

Normal sectoral sono-probes are too big and will not have a high resolution at greater depths. Together with the endoscope, or freehand, the ENS-catheter can be placed at each target through a 2-mm gap or channel, leaving enough space for instrumentation.

The imaging geometry of the transnasal approach is a frontal scan that is orthogonal to the endoscope shaft at the tip of the endoscope (Figs. 2.63–2.72).

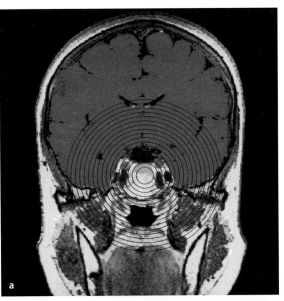

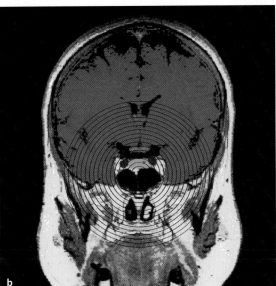

Fig. 2.63a–g. Frontal MR scans of pituitary region. The cranial MR slices are reconstructed in color and show pituitary gland (*green*), tumor (*violet*), carotid artery (*red*), optic system (*orange*), brain (*blue*), and surrounding tissue (*yellow*) of skull. Penetrating with the sono-catheter transsphenoidally, the sellar region is imaged by the scan, which represents the typical structure. The sono-wave is shown schematically, coming close to the sella on the floor of the third ventricle

2

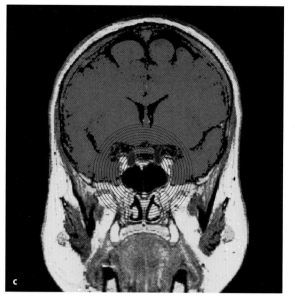

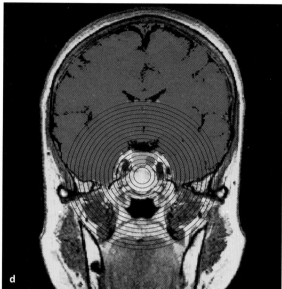

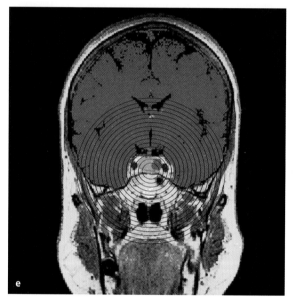

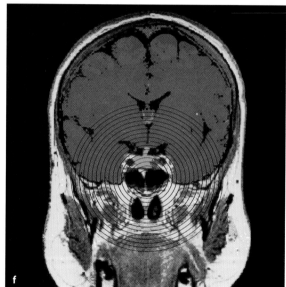

Fig. 2.63c–g

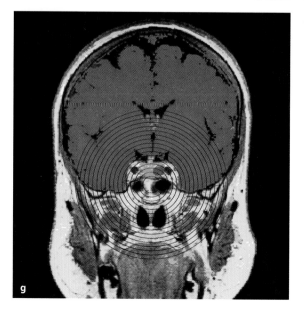

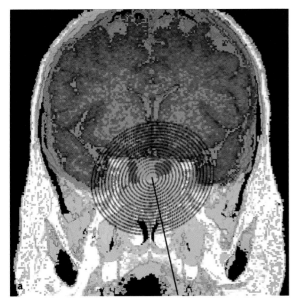

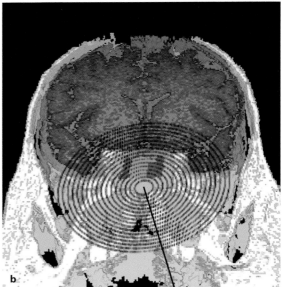

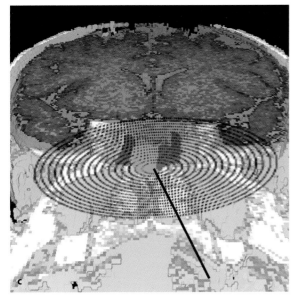

Fig. 2.64a–c. Frontal 3D slices of MR at different inclinations. A sequence of several MR slices is reconstructed in 3D and presented in color, showing pituitary gland (*green*), tumor (*violet*), carotid artery (*red*), brain (*blue*), and surrounding tissue (*yellow*). The imaging plane of the sono-catheter depends on the steepness of the angle at which the endoscope is inserted transnasally

2

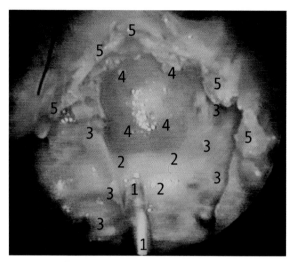

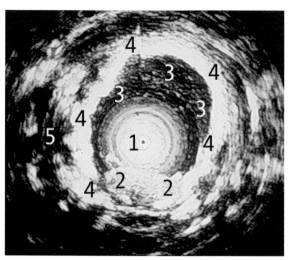

Fig. 2.65. Sella, transnasal. The endoscope is introduced pernasally into the sphenoid sinus with a typical surface, and the sono-probe (*1*) is placed on the floor of the sella (*2*). Lateral to the sella (*2*) the impression of the carotid artery (*3*) is visible. In the deep tissue, the dorsal wall of this large sphenoidal sinus (clivus) (*4*) is present. The cutting edge of the sinus wall (*5*) surrounds the bony cavity

Fig. 2.66. Sella, transnasal scan. The sono-probe (*1*) is located in the sphenoid sinus (*3*) and touching the sella within the pituitary gland (*2*). The bony wall of the sphenoid sinus (*4*) is clearly visible, as is one cavernous sinus (*5*)

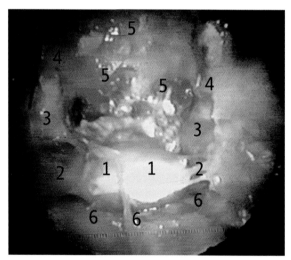

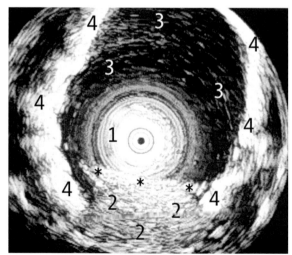

Fig. 2.67. Dura of sella, transnasal. After bone resection, the endoscope is directed at the dural surface of the sella (*1*) with the typical hypophyseal ligament (*2*). The cavernous sinus is open on both sides, and the carotid artery (*3*) inside is visible up to the petrous apex (*4*). The clivus (*5*) is lower than the sphenoid sinus and is not resected

Fig. 2.68. Dura of sella, transnasal scan. The sono-probe (*1*) is in contact with the sellar dura (*), while the pituitary gland is visible (*2*). The sphenoid sinus cavity (*3*) is marked by bone (*4*)

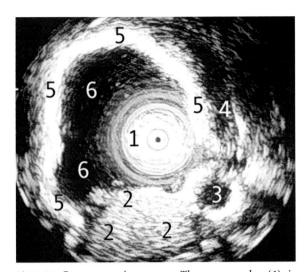

Fig. 2.69. Cavernous sinus scan. The sono-probe (1) is inside the sphenoid sinus (6) and attached to the dura of the sella with the pituitary gland (2) and to the cavernous sinus (4) with the carotid artery (3). The bony wall (5) of the sphenoid sinus is clearly visible

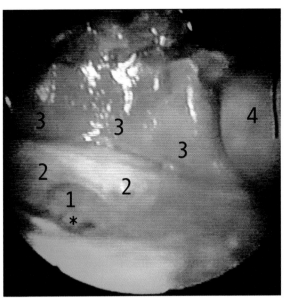

Fig. 2.70. Diaphragm of sella, transnasal. The endoscope is placed in the empty sella. After resection of pituitary gland, only the dissected stalk (*) within the hiatus (1) of the diaphragm (2) and the naked bony dorsum of the sella (3) become visible. The carotid artery (4) is in close contact with the dorsum of the sella

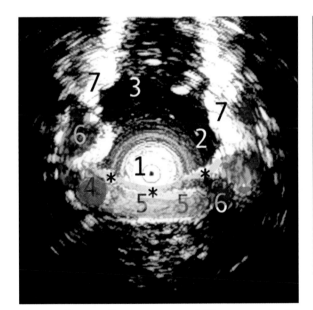

Fig. 2.71. Empty sella scan, transnasal. The sono-probe (1) is inside the empty sella (2) and is then pushed further toward the diaphragm of sella (*). Caudally the sphenoid sinus (3) is visible with its bony wall (7), and lateral to the sella (2), the cavernous sinus (6) with, on the *left side*, the carotid artery (4). Inside the empty sella (2) the sono-probe visualizes the optic chiasm (5)

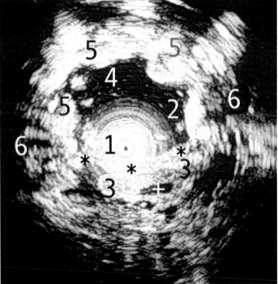

Fig. 2.72. Optic chiasm scan, transnasal. The sono-probe (1) is positioned in the empty sella (2) and then pushed against the diaphragm of the sella (*), visualizing the optic chiasm (3) and the supraoptic recess (+). The cavernous sinus (6) is visible laterally and below the bony wall (5) of the sphenoid sinus (4)

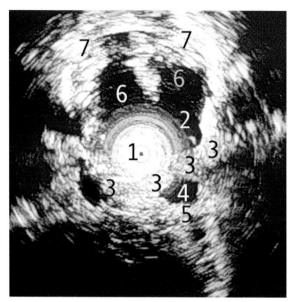

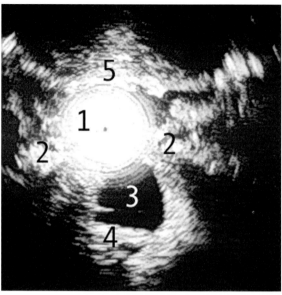

Fig. 2.73. Optic chiasm and third ventricle scan, transnasal. The sono-probe (1) is now in the empty sella (2), so that the optic chiasm (3) is visualized through the diaphragm and it is possible to see into the third ventricle with the supraoptic recess (4) and the anterior commissure (5). Caudally the sphenoid sinus (6) and the bone of the clivus (7) are visible

Fig. 2.74. Third ventricle scan, transnasal. The sono-probe (1) is pushed against the dorsum of the sella (5) and the diaphragm within the empty sella, visualizing the optic tracts (2) plus the anterior third ventricle (3) with the anterior commissure (4)

Summary Remarks on ENS Anatomy

Imaging of the *ventricular system* by ENS is very clear and has a precise shape that is easily recognized, giving good orientation. The *basal cisterns* and the subarachnoid space are also clearly visible. This is due to the echo-difference between CSF and neural tissue. Therefore, all parts surrounded by CSF can be precisely represented and changes in size and shifting are reliably detected.

Dural structures such as the falx cerebri or the tentorium appear with a strong echo signal that makes them useful for orientation.

Of course, all *bony structures* give a high-echo signal and are detected even when the parenchyma is already outside the detecting depth. The skull borders will be shown on the display even when the parenchyma is only present in a 2-cm radius around the probe.

Vessels give a higher signal than the neural tissue, but will be recognized in clinical use even better from the clear appearance of the blood flow and pulsation.

The *choroid plexus* also has a strong signal, showing up even the finest villi spreading in the same way as fingers, which can be seen during clinical application of the technique as movements due to the irrigation of the endoscope and pulsation of the vessels. The different fibers and nuclei of *neural tissue* do not show up distinctly.

Since ultrasound imaging is in real time and on-line, it can detect all such changes in the anatomy as size of ventricles, shifting of tissue, pulsation of liquids, and movements of the displayed sonoprobe itself. All this means that the movements of the endoscope within the anatomy are visible in the sono-scan leading to the specific *neuronavigation* characteristic (see CD-ROM). Neuronavigation has become a major topic in actual neurosurgery regarding numerous publications. Some authors even believe that it could change Yasargil's concept of the subarachnoid approach (Wurm et al. 2000; Yasargil 1994a–c).

However, despite all efforts, intraoperative CT and MR have not yet reached online and real-time characteristics. Only X-ray and sonography fulfill the navigation requirements of real-time feedback. Sonography can moreover be used as an online technique without negative side effects.

Training in sonography is necessary before some of the difficulties in interpretation of the images can be mastered (Makuuchi et al. 1998Sutcliffe 1991). If endosonography is not to lead to frustration it is most important to learn how to get a competent image. The first step will be to know the imaging characteristics of the anatomical structures so as to be aware of what to expect and what the typical features of an anatomical structure look like in the endosonographic scan. Therefore, this work was started with anatomical examinations. The next step was to learn how to adjust the image of the sono-scan in terms of orientation, frequency, and zoom.

The benefits of sonography have already been documented (Auer et al. 1988; Auer and van Velthoven 1990; Sutcliffe 1991; Van Velthoven and Auer 1990), The benefits of endosonography will be confirmed as time goes on, but depend primarily on the user's patience in following the above steps (see also chap. 3). Experience is limited as yet, but has shown that these are essential.

Precise imaging quality and correct adjustment are indispensable for neuronavigation by ENS. Clinical examples (chap. 3; for video clips see chap. 4) will show what can be done and which problems can be solved or at least simplified.

In summary, tests of transendoscopic sonography catheters have shown interesting *imaging* and *neuronavigation* qualities:

- Precise imaging of anatomical structures
- Ability to 'see' into the parenchyma
- An axial overview: 'mini-CT' (in addition to endoscopic viewing)
- Compensation of 'blind angles' of the endoscope
- Compensation of problems that can hamper vision, such as bleeding, no space, dirty lens, technical pitfalls
- Real-time imaging for neuronavigation 'brain radar'
- Online observation of all movements and physical changes (size of ventricles, shift of tissue, blood flow, pulsation)

2

A *preliminary list of indications* can be derived from the above:

Indication	Reason for using ENS
Ventricular puncture	Subependymal target
Fenestration of cysts	Small ventricles, intraparenchymal
Tumor biopsy	Targeting
Examination of aneurysm	Neck, rupture side, pulsation, etc.
Morphometric ICP online monitoring	Ventricular size and change
CT substitute in ICU	Online monitoring of ICH, edema, etc.
Endoneuronavigation	Real time, simple, not expensive

This list seems to be worth examination to determine when application of this technique is appropriate.

Handling is easy, once competence is acquired, as is integration of the technique into the endoscopic process. The equipment is mobile, small, and quite inexpensive relative to that needed for other navigation and intraoperative imaging techniques.

In conclusion, it is apparent from the studies that ENS warrants large-scale clinical testing now that the boundary conditions are documented and the application process has been elaborated. Past experience of its clinical usage is documented as detailed below in chap. 3.

Clinical Application

3

Contents

Materials and Methods

Intraoperative endoneurosonographic (ENS) imagings prepared during surgery on 52 selected patients between April 1996 and July 2000 were examined. There were 23 female and 29 male patients, and their mean age was 42 (2–69) years. In most cases Aloka (Aloka Deutschland, Düsseldorf, Germany) sono equipment was used because equipment supplied by this company had yielded superior imaging results in

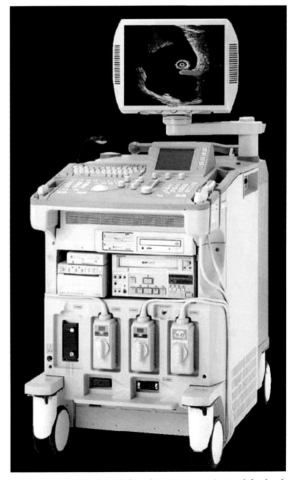

Fig. 3.1. The ALOKA Highend ENS system is used for both general and transendoscopic sonography. On the display seen here, for example, a scan of the 3d ventricle with the sono-probe is in touch with interthalamic mass

Objective

After transendoscopic sono-catheters had been tested in the laboratory for imaging characteristics and practicability (chap. 2), clinical application was then studied with special reference to imaging and navigation capabilities, practicability, safety, and preliminary indications.

The questions were whether the promising results of the laboratory work would be confirmed and the practicability in operative routine be satisfactory; what problems might show up and what problems needed to be resolved; and, finally, what limits there might be on their use in clinical practice.

the laboratory. The technical specifications are listed in Chapter 1. Today, transendoscopic sonography is integrated in a highend machine made by Aloka, which makes it possible to substitute and compare transendoscopic sonography and general sonography easily in the same cases (Fig 3.1).

Because of additional safety precautions concerned with sterilization, in 25 selected cases a short perioperative antibiotic prophylaxis was administered.

This work with patients differed from the laboratory work in that two sizes (diameters) of catheters were used: 6-F catheters for transendoscopic use and 8-F catheters for freehand use, whether paraendoscopically or without endoscopy at all. In such cases an 8-F catheter was used as a 'sono-dissector.'

Results

Ergonomics in the Operating Room (see chap. 5)

The sono equipment does not take up a lot of space. The machine itself was placed outside the sterile area, and a nurse handed the long thin catheter to the surgeon to be fixed near the patient's head. This meant that the equipment did not in any way hamper the operating procedure or the surgeon's movements. Preparation of the equipment took only minutes, with some differences between the two systems used. The sono system was easier to prepare than an endoscope.

As the catheter was inserted in the working channel, use of the endoscope was not obstructed. When used freehand, the sono-catheter is comparable with a dissector in terms of handling and of space requirements. Therefore, it was possible to direct the catheter even in small deep gaps to obtain optimal imaging. If there were any problems with imaging quality decreasing as a function of known distance (as is known with macro sono-probes), these were not apparent.

From the ergonomics viewpoint the head-mounted display (HMD) system was helpful, enabling the display of several items of imaging information at once and being in the optimal position at all times regardless of the surgeon's head position. This was ideal for ENS, as the endoscopic image and the sono-picture were always presented together, making correlation of the images and navigation easier and safer (Figs. 3.2, 3.3).

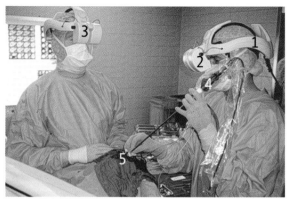

Fig. 3.2. The HMD system. The head-mounted display system (1) allows multiple imaging information to be displayed on one screen in an ergonomic working position. The surgeon sees all information displayed directly at eye level (2 and 3), regardless of his/her head position, and is free to concentrate on the endoscope (4) and the patient's head (5). The assistant can follow the procedure even without a monitor and in a position that is helpful for performance of the procedure regardless of the monitor's position. The kind of information displayed can be changed and selected by voice control. With this system the surgeon can perform time-consuming procedures while maintaining a relaxed position and a high level of concentration

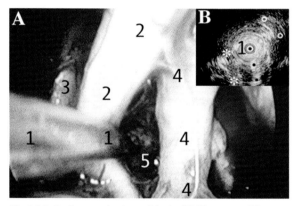

Fig. 3.3A, B. Surgeon's view with the HMD system. The surgeon's views of the information presented by the endoscope (A) and by the sono-scan (B) are both real time and online in parallel. The endoscopic view controls the sono-probe optically (A1) and the sono-scan, sonographically (B1). The sono-probe (A1+B1) is positioned between the right optic nerve (2) and the right carotid artery (4) in the retrosellar area (5). In the field that was previously not visible, the sonographic view (B) represents the left carotid artery (* *) and the right carotid artery (° °) plus a remnant of a calcified craniopharyngioma (. .). The parallel presentation of both images on one screen regardless of head position makes working and correlation of the two images much easier

General Remarks and List of Lesions

In clinical use the sono-catheter has superior imaging and navigation abilities to those seen in anatomical laboratory work. Real-time and online characteristics represent changes such as shifting, pulsation, CSF flow, and changes in size and form of structures. When confronted with clinical problems, this technique still has some limitations. The sono-catheter has nevertheless proved to be a valuable tool for sorting out unresolved problems and to be much easier to use than other instruments. Moreover, there appears to be an interesting potential for further developments.

Thus, the sono-catheter has been tested intraoperatively in imaging of a variety of lesions (Table 3.1).

Ventricles. The easiest application was *navigation of the endoscope into the ventricles*. The catheter was inserted into the working channel of the endoscope, and after the endoscope had penetrated into the brain the catheter was pushed ahead, scanning the area in front of the endoscope. The falx cerebri was used for orientation; the sono-scan first had to be adjusted to the anatomical orientation based on the falx cerebri and also adjusted to the endoscope's view. Once this had been accomplished, the catheter functioned as a scanning tool and literally spoke, acting in the same way as a 'seeing' Cushing cannula. Once the typical shapes of the ventricles were on the display the catheter could be used as a guide along which the scope was advanced into the ventricle without loss of any cerebrospinal fluid (CSF). This strategy was helpful in small ventricles, where punctures were made in unusual positions, and also in ventricles displaced by edema, hematomas, tumors, or congenital lesions.

Another use in the ventricular system was for assistance in *third ventriculocisternostomy*. Various changes to the ventricles, and especially to the floor of the third ventricle, can make it difficult, if not impossible, to target the perforation point. In such cases the sono-catheter can be used for blunt perforation. Before the endoscope sees the features of the interpeduncular cistern, the scan of the sono-probe will show the dorsum sellae, the prime landmark, on the display. This can be used to adjust the sono-scan orientation if necessary. The next most important landmark will be the basilar artery, but the tentorial notch, the oculomotor nerve, and the ventral surface and parenchyma of the midbrain are also discernable. All these structures can be used for orientation and navigation, and they can be perceived while still invisible to the endoscope. In many cases the infundibulum was deep enough to allow visualization of parts or all of the circle of Willis, and of the blood flow inside its vessels.

When there are problems with visualization the possibility of damaging these structures is markedly increased, and measures must be taken to ensure that the risk is managed in an acceptable manner (Table 3.2).

Table 3.1. Lesions

Type of lesion	n
Ventricular lesions	20
Cystic lesions	9
Intracerebral hematoma	5
Tumor	15
Hypohyseal tumor (transnasal)	6
Aneurysm	6
Trigeminal neuralgia	1
HIV/granuloma	1
Cavernoma	1

Table 3.2. Ventricular lesions

Type of ventricular lesion	Action taken	n
Hydrocephalus	Catheter placement	2
Colloid cyst	Viscosity?	2
Hematoma	Communication with foramen of Monro	3
Ventriculitis	Navigated septostomy	1
Aqueduct stenosis	Third ventriculostomy (ETV)	6
Velum interpositum cyst	Fenestration to ventricle	2
Cyst	Multiple stomies, orientation	2
Tumor	Borders, shift, targeting, remnants	5

Nonshunted ETV Cases

Case 1

Clinical History

This 41-year-old woman had a delayed recovery after a hysterectomy. She complained of constant fatigue, slowness in moving and thinking, and memory disturbance. Her gait looked parkinsonoid, but she was continent for urine and micturition was normal. There was a slight dysmetria and bradydiadochokinesis.

CT showed three-ventricular hydrocephalus with no edema. MR showed an arachnoid cyst below the quadrigeminal lamina and above the upper cerebellar vermis, where the superior medullary velum was impairing flow through the aqueduct (Fig. 3.4).

Treatment and Outcome

On 15 April 1996 a first endoscopic third ventriculostomy (ETV) was done using ENS imaging (Figs. 3.5–3.11). The floor of the third ventricle was transparent and very thin, giving adequate sight of anatomical structures of the interpeduncular cistern and the sellar region (Fig. 3.9). However, as the first small perforation was made, the membranous tissue started to move with the CSF, and all the anatomical landmarks mentioned above ceased to be visible. The imaging with the ENS catheter had to be correlated with anatomical landmarks before

the perforation was made; these were still present afterwards, allowing suitable navigation (Fig. 3.11). Various levels of the pathway of ETV represented typical features already known from the work in the anatomy laboratory (Figs. 3.6, 3.8, 3.11). The clinical imaging was characterized by stronger contrast than was seen during the anatomy laboratory experience.

The postoperative course was uncomplicated, and the patient went home 7 days after her operation. MR control showed a decrease in ventricular size, and the patient was free of her earlier symptoms (Fig 3.4).

The theoretical variation in the angle of approach was limited by the size of the foramen of Monro and the diameter of the endoscope, resulting in an optimal situation for the approach angle.

The necessity for additional turning of the endoscope depended on the angle of the light aperture and the distance of the endoscope from the target. With widening lens aperture and increasing distance between endoscope and target the necessity for turning the endoscope away from the primary approach angle lessened. An angled lens could also have been used to avoid angling the scope.

ENS defines how far away an invisible target is and how much additional turning of the endoscope is required (Figs. 3.4–3.11).

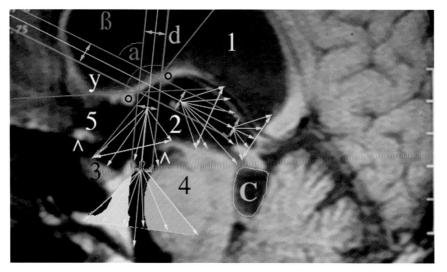

Fig. 3.4. Aqueduct stenosis. In this case, a cystic lesion (*C/orange*) caused an aqueduct stenosis with hydrocephalus of lateral (*1*) and third (*2*) ventricles. Bulging of infundibular recess towards the pituitary gland (*3*) and the supra-optic recess (*5*) with depression of optic chiasm (∧) and floor of third ventricle (∧). The foramen of Monro (° °) is enlarged

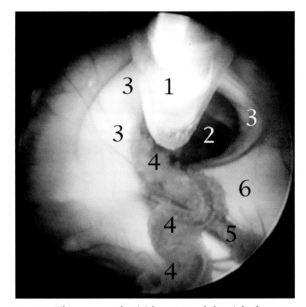

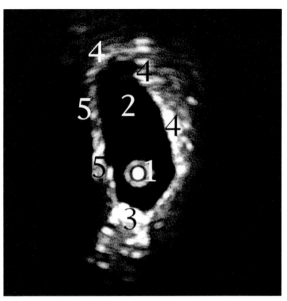

Fig. 3.5. The sono-probe (*1*) has entered the right foramen of Monro (*2*) formed by the fornix (*3*) and the choroid plexus (*4*). The thalamostriate vein (*5*) is crossing the lamina affixa (*6*). The tip of the probe (*1*) can be accurately controlled by the endoscope and can be pushed ahead into the working channel of the endoscope, independently visualizing parts that are invisible to the endoscope

Fig. 3.6. The sono-probe (*1*) is located in the right foramen of Monro (*2*) formed by the fornix (*4*) and the choroid plexus (*3*). The scan represents the pellucid septum (*5*)

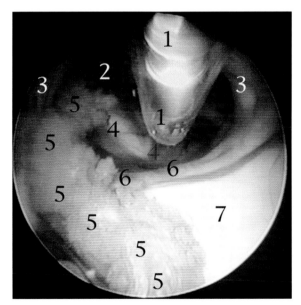

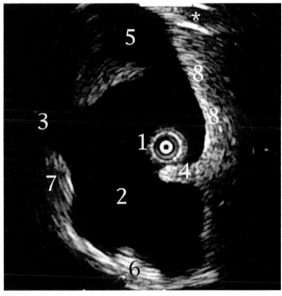

Fig. 3.7. The sono-probe (*1*) is pushed into the foramen of Monro (*2*) formed by the fornix (*3*) touching the intermediate mass (*4*). The choroid plexus (*5*) is crossing the small 'foraminal' vein (*6*) and the lamina affixa (*7*)

Fig. 3.8. The sono-probe (*1*) scan is now showing a semi-axial view of the third ventricle (*2*) and its own position (*1*) in the anatomy. It has made contact with the intermediate mass (*4*) and is close to the fornix (*8*). The choroid plexus (*4*) of the roof is visible, as are the contralateral foramen of Monro (*3*) and thalamus (*7*). Through the lamina terminalis at the supraoptic recess (*5*) the anterior cerebral artery (***) is scanned. The ependymal border of the ventricle can be delineated exactly

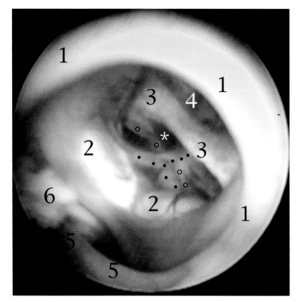

Fig. 3.9 The sono-probe has now been drawn back into the working channel and the endoscope gives a good view of the floor of the third ventricle. The endoscope is approaching the foramen of Monro on the right side formed by the fornix (*1*). The sono-scan shows the right frontal horn (*1*), pellucid septum (*2*), and choroid plexus (*3*). The view is directed to the floor of the third ventricle with mamillary bodies (*2*), the dorsum of the sella (*3*), the diaphragm of the sella (*4*), and the basilar (...) artery and its division into P1 (...) and SuCA (°°°). The translucent membrane of the bulging caudal infundibular recess covers the landmark structures (***)

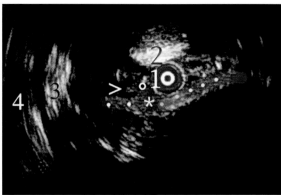

Fig. 3.11. After perforation of the floor of the third ventricle by the sono-probe (*1*), the dorsum of the sella (*2*) becomes visible in the sono-scan. This is one of the main sono-landmarks, near which we see the basilar head (***) with both P1 segments (....) and the basilar trunk (°) and left SuCA (>). As the sono tip (*1*) itself is visible, it can be exactly navigated, as can the endoscope. The blood flow can be seen on the monitor (or video)

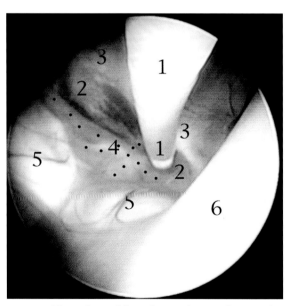

Fig. 3.10. The catheter (*1*) perforates the membranous infundibular recess (*2*) just behind the dorsum of the sella (*3*) and lateral to the basilar head (*4*) with its branches (...). Mamillary bodies (*5*) and the thalamus (*6*) are visible

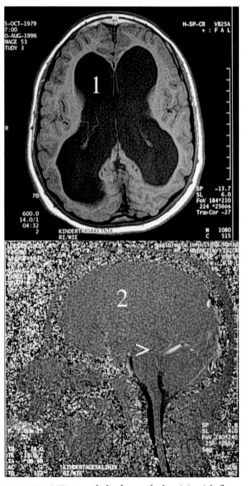

Fig. 3.12. MR reveals hydrocephalus (*1*) with flow-sensitive sequences; there is no flow void signal in the aqueduct (>)

Case 2

Clinical History

This young man aged 19 years had undergone an ETV 2 years previously for treatment of obstructive hydrocephalus. His cerebral spastic behavior subsequently took a better course. Slowly, however, the condition stagnated and eventually symptoms of elevated intracranial pressure (ICP) became obvious, with headache and coordination problems.

Treatment and Outcome

MR did not reveal a flow signal compatible with an open stoma on the floor of the third ventricle (Fig. 3.12, 3.13). During surgery not the slightest sign of a previous ventriculostomy was found on the floor of the third ventricle. ENS (Fig. 3.14) was used in addition to control the imaging (Fig. 3.15) by supplying two-fold images yielded by endoscopy and sonography, and its end-effect was comparable with that of MR and neuronavigation data. It was possible to demonstrate excellent vascular real-time imaging and several landmark structures around the sella (Figs. 3.16–3.20). ENS control was continued while a ventriculocisternostomy was carried out, and no additional membrane was found at a deep level.

Postoperatively the man did well: motor function was developing much better and spasticity decreased, as did tremor. Six months later a clinical check-up examination showed no symptoms of raised ICP. but motor function was worsening again and MR control did not confirm a patent flow signal. Unfortunately, the patient was lost to follow-up and the clinical history therefore ends at this point. Continuous ICP monitoring was planned, but has not so far been possible. It must be assumed that a relevant resorption deficit is involved.

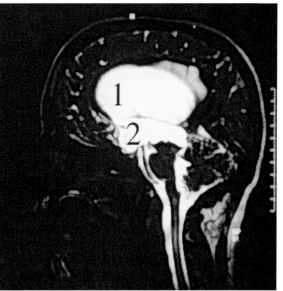

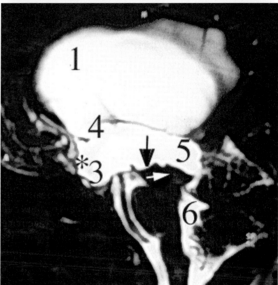

Fig. 3.13. Again the CISS sequences show massive hydrocephalus of the lateral (*1*) and third (*2*) ventricles and a great deal of additional detail. The foramen of Monro (*4*) is enlarged, and the supraoptic recess (*), infundibular recess (*3*), and pineal recess (*5*) are bulging. The roof of the midbrain (*downward arrow*) is pressed caudally; no aqueduct is visible (*arrow to right*); and the fourth ventricle is normal in size (*6*)

3

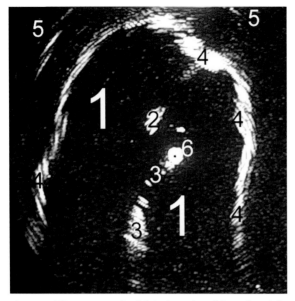

Fig. 3.14. The sono-probe (*6*) is introduced into the right lateral ventricle, showing both lateral ventricles (*1*) in contact with the right-sided choroid plexus (*3*). Remnants of the falx cerebri (*2*) and the CSF–ependymal border (*4*) are visible and hyperdense at this low zoom; even the skull (*5*) is scanned

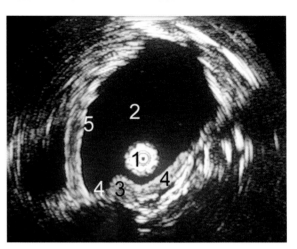

Fig. 3.16. The sono-probe (*1*) is now introduced into the third ventricle (*2*) deep in the caudally bulging floor, causing a scanning plane at the level of the circle of Willis (*red*). The basilar artery (*3*) is seen, and both P1 (*4*) and left Pcom (*5*) are visible

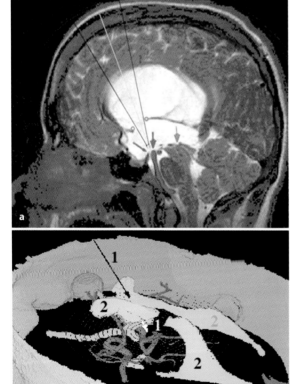

Fig. 3.15 a, b. Image processing can give a most attractive presentation of information with stronger contrast: A Basilar artery (*red* ⇓) is pushing the floor of the third ventricle cranially, not allowing the typical downward bulging of the floor. The aqueduct is stenotic (*violet* ⇓). The distance between the dorsum of the sella (*blue arrow*) and the basilar artery (*red* ⇓) for ETV (*black* ↓) through the foramen of Monro (° °) is very small. The sono-catheter (*yellow* ↓) can be placed in the infundibular recess, since it is able to scan (*yellow* ↔) the vessels of the circle of Willis. B With the aid of an ENS catheter (*1* ↓ *black, white*) with sono-wave (()), vessels can be seen quite well through the ventricular system because of their blood flow, which is invisible to the endoscope

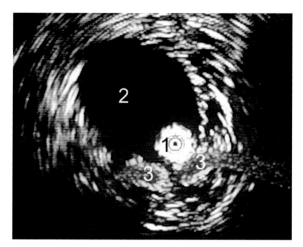

Fig. 3.17. The sono-probe (*1*) has penetrated deep into the third ventricle (*2*) and the caudal bulging infundibular recess close to the basilar artery and is scanning the division in both P1 segments (*3/red*)

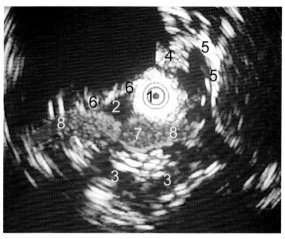

Fig. 3.18. The sono-probe (*1*) is now pushed into the infundibular recess (*2*), which appears as a membrane (*6*). It makes contact with the dorsum of the sella (*4*) and the basilar artery (*7*), while branching to both SuCAs (*8*). The tentorial notch (*5*) and the pons (*3*) are also visible

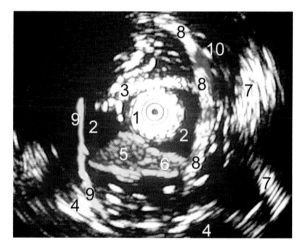

Fig. 3.19. The sono-probe (*1*) is placed deep into the infundibular recess (*2*), touching the dorsum of the sella (*3*) and the basilar artery (*5*), where the SuCA (*6*) branches. Right (*8*) and left oculomotor (*9*) nerves are scanned, running from the mesencephalon (*4*) through the cavernous sinus (*10*). The tentorium (*7*) is coming into view on the right

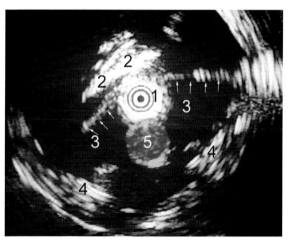

Fig. 3.20. The sono-probe (*1*) has perforated the floor of the third ventricle and is pushed into the interpeduncular cistern (*3*), touching the clivus (*2*) and the basilar artery (*5*). The arachnoid wall of the cistern (*arrows*) is clearly visible. Dorsally, the border of the pons (*4*) is present

Case 3

Clinical History

This 8-year-old girl presented with a 3-week history of headache and with a diagnosis of neurofibromatosis (I), which was known also to be present in several other members of her family (brother, mother, and grandmother). An urgent MR showed internal hydrocephalus (Fig. 3.21) with aqueduct stenosis and periventricular edema; several lesions related to the neurofibromatosis were already known.

Treatment and Outcome

An ENS-controlled ventriculocisternostomy showed all vessels in the circle of Willis (Figs. 3.22, 3.23). After the ETV the symptoms disappeared, none of the changes caused by the hydrocephalus being seen on an MR 12 hours after the operation (Fig. 3.24). The girl went home on the 7th day after surgery.

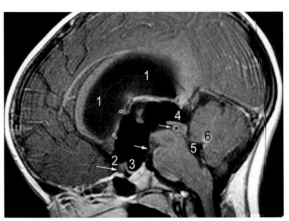

Fig. 3.21. This is a typical MR of a patient with an aqueductal stenosis (*smaller arrows*). Occlusive hydrocephalus of lateral (*1*) and third ventricles, with enlarged foramen of Monro (° °), wide open infundibular (*3*), supraoptic (*2*), and pineal recesses (*4*), and bulging floor of the third ventricle. The entrance to the aqueduct (*small arrow to right*) is wide open because of the caudal position of the stenosis, while the optic chiasm (*long arrow to right*) is pre-fixed

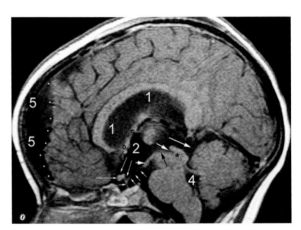

Fig. 3.22. Postoperative MR next day shows that all patho logic changes seen in Fig. 3.21 have disappeared. The aqueduct stenosis (→) caused by a small tumor (*) is of course still visible. Lateral (*1*) and third (*2*) ventricles and foramen of Monro (° °) are much smaller, and the infundibular (↓), supraoptic (↓), and pineal recesses (→) are narrow again. The floor of the third ventricle (↑), the mamillary body, and the roof of the mesencephalon (↑), like the pituitary stalk (→) and optic chiasm (→), have regained their normal positions. The fourth ventricle (*4*) is unchanged and some air is visible (*5*) postoperatively

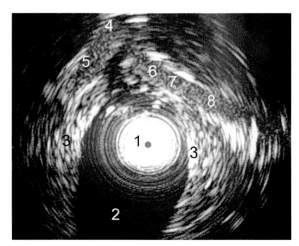

Fig. 3.23. The sono-probe (*1*) is in the anterior third ventricle (*2*). On the way to the infundibulum the sonograph shows vessels (*red*) that are invisible to the endoscope. Left ICA (*4*), M1 segment (*5*), A1 segment (*6*), ACA (*7*), and right A1 (*8*) with blood flow are visible. The thalami (*3*) on both sides can be seen (*3*)

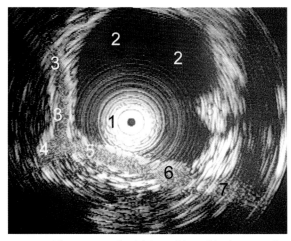

Fig. 3.24. The sono-probe (*1*) is positioned in the posterior third ventricle (*2*). Through the walls, it shows the left PcoA (*3*), P2 (*4*), and P1 (*5*) segments, the basilar tip (*6*), the right P1 () segment, and the blood flow in all vessels

Preshunted ETV Cases

Case 4

Clinical History

This little 3-year-old girl had recurrent infections and shunt infections, having been primarily shunted because of a communicating posthemorrhage hydrocephalus present at birth. After several shunt revisions she suffered a shunt-related ileus. Because of the risk of infection, the pediatric specialists did not recommend a VA shunt.

The child was admitted with a query as to whether an endoscopic procedure would be possible. Careful analysis of all the neuroradiological pictures taken since the onset of her illness gave rise to the suspicion of an obstructive component, especially in view of the history of infection.

However, there were three classic contraindications for ETV: communicating hydrocephalus, a posthemorrhagic cause of hydrocephalus, and multiple infections. Figure 3.25 shows plain radiographs on which the shunt system is seen in its typical location on (1) lateral and (2) a-p views.

Treatment and Outcome

The pediatricians urged us to find a solution that would not involve the risks inherent in shunt procedures; the usual treatment with implantation of a shunt had already failed several times, with a high risk of complications. In addition, an obstructive component of the patient's hydrocephalus was playing a part, and we hoped it would be possible to deal with it by the endoscopic approach. In short, it seemed that despite the contraindications mentioned above there was no better chance of saving the patient, and we therefore decided to proceed with ETV. After ETV, which showed significant changes to the subarachnoid cisterns and the ependyma, and after explantation of the shunt an extracranial drain was left in place for ICP measurement. The patient did not have raised ICP, but there were problems caused by a CSF fistula. After removal of the drain lumbar drainage was accomplished by means of internal fistulation by lumbar puncture and the subgaleal fistula was closed with a fat graft. With this step-by-step strategy the CSF system slowly adapted to self-regulation within 3 weeks. The girl is now shunt free, and her clinical condition is good.

Because of the earlier long-term shunting the ventricles were small. Therefore, in this case the usual technical solution of neuronavigation was applied, which gave us the opportunity to combine neuronavigation with ENS (Figs. 3.26–3.29).

3

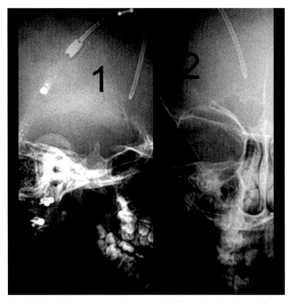

Fig. 3.25. A shunt system in a typical location is shown here on plain radiographs from lateral (*1*) and a-p (*2*) views

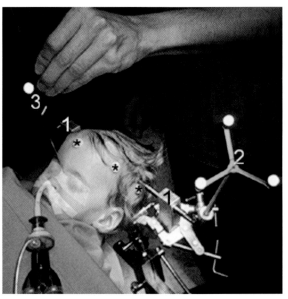

Fig. 3.26. When neuronavigation is to be used various essential steps must precede the planned operation. The head must be fixed completely in a holding device (*1*) and equipped with a target arm (*2*). A pointer (*3*) makes it possible to reference the head at the markers (*) with the navigation system

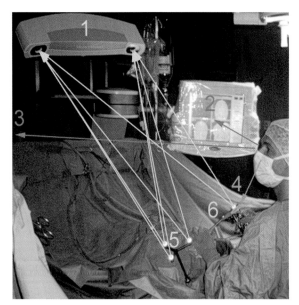

Fig. 3.27. Neuronavigation setting in the operating room needs a special geometry to function. The view for the camera (*1*) must not be hampered by the target arm (*5*) or the endoscope (*6*). The surgeon must be able to see the navigation monitor (*2*) and the endoscope monitor (*3*) together at the same time and somehow integrate all the data from both while also coordinating the manipulations and adapting to the spatial and neuropsychological conditions of neuronavigated endoscopy

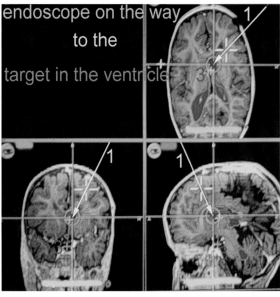

endoscope on the way
to the
target in the ventricle

Fig. 3.28. The endoscope (*1*) has now been navigated into the frontal horn of the right lateral ventricle (*2*). The target point (*3*) is the interpeduncular cistern. There is a difference of more than 10 mm between the navigation image and the endoscopic image. When the tip (*cross*) of the endoscope (*1*) has reached the ventricular target in the right frontal horn (*2*) the endoscope monitor still shows the parenchyma of the white matter because there was only a slight loss of CSF on puncture and because the ependyma, which was pushed by the lens before being torn, is so elastic

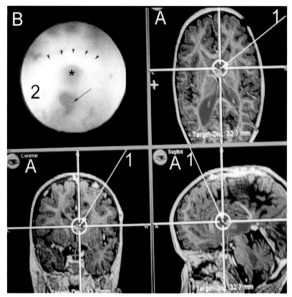

Fig. 3.29. The endoscope (*1*) has reached the frontal horn (*blue*) on the navigation display (*white cross*), but the endoscopic view (*B*) shows the real position of the endoscope in the third ventricle (*2*). The typical appearance of the floor (*2*) has changed, and the optic chiasm (↓), infundibular recess (*), and infundibulum (←) are hardly visible. The difference between the navigation position (*A*) and the endoscopic, real, position (*B*) was more than 10 mm in this case

Several steps were necessary before the operation to make neuronavigation possible:

■ On the day before the procedure, markers were put on the child's head and additional shaving was necessary (Fig. 3.26).
■ An extra 3D MR or CT when these markers in place was necessary.
■ Data had to be imported, and computer-assisted planning was needed (Fig. 3,27).
■ The child's head had to be fixed in a sharp headrest(Fig. 3.26).
■ The headrest had to be equipped with a target arm (Fig.3 26).
■ After positioning and starting, the navigation system was adjusted by means of a pointer (Fig. 3.26).
■ The geometry of all components had to be applied to the needs of the navigation system (Fig. 3.27).

This list illustrates some of the typical problems encountered in the process of neuronavigation (Figs. 3. 26–3.29).

The neuronavigation setup in the operating room needs a special geometry to function. The camera's view must not be blocked by the target arm or the endoscope. The surgeon needs to watch the navigation monitor and the endoscope monitor at the same time. Somehow, he or she has to integrate all the data from both and also to coordinate the manipulations in such a way as to suit the spatial and neuropsychological conditions of neuronavigated endoscopy. A situation of this kind can be regarded as an ergonomic trauma for the surgeon (see Figs. 3.26, 3.27; chap. 5).

In Fig. 3.28 the endoscope has been navigated into the frontal horn of the right lateral ventricle. The target point is the interpeduncular cistern. There is a difference of more than 10 mm between the navigation image and the endoscopic image. When the tip of the endoscope has reached the ventricular target in the right frontal horn the endoscope monitor still shows the parenchyma of the white matter. This is because little CSF was lost at the time of puncture and because the ependyma, which is pushed by the lens before being torn, is so elastic.

Figure 3.29 shows the endoscope when it has reached the frontal horn on the navigation display, but the endoscopic view shows its real position, which is in the third ventricle. The typical appearance of the floor has changed, and the optic chiasm, infundibular recess, and infundibulum are hardly visible. There was more than 10 mm between the navigation position (Fig. 3.29A) and the real position shown in the endoscopic display (Fig. 3.29B). In Fig. 3.30 the endoscope is shown as it is advanced along the clivus into the prepontine cistern at the level where the AICA branches off from the basilar artery. There are strong arachnoid adhesions between the cisternal wall and the basilar artery. This view was achieved only by endoscopic control and was not possible by navigation. In the case of lack of vision it becomes dangerous even to leave the area at times, because the navigation image is not a real-time image.

As As an experienced surgeon relies more heavily on anatomy than on navigation systems, the outcome in this case was excellent. Figure 3.31 shows the child the day after the ETV, and she is already reading. The only pain she complained of was that caused by the positioning screws on the headrest.

3

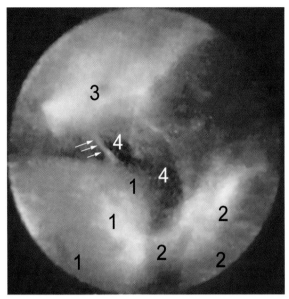

Fig. 3.30. The endoscope is advanced along the clivus (*3*) into the prepontine cistern (*4*) at the level where the AICA (*2*) is branching from the basilar artery (*1*). There are strong arachnoid adhesions (→) between cisternal wall and basilar artery (*1*). This view could only be achieved by endoscopic control and not by navigation. If vision is lost, even leaving the area becomes dangerous at times, because the navigation image is not real time

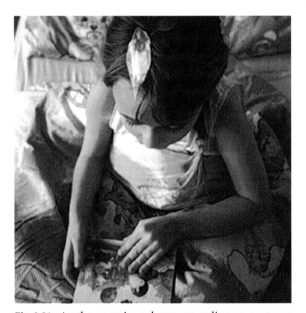

Fig. 3.31. As the experienced surgeon relies on anatomy more than on navigation systems, the case shown in Figs. 3.28–3.30 had an excellent outcome. The child is seen here on the day after ETV and is already reading. The only pain she complained of was that resulting from the positioning screws of the headrest

Case 5

Clinical History

This 9-year-old girl had been shunted earlier because of hydrocephalus and was admitted this time with a 4-week history of headache and intermittent vomiting. The shunt system did not show any irregularities after diagnosis. MR (Fig. 3.32) revealed asymmetrical hydrocephalus with the right lateral ventricle small and the left one enlarged. A meticulous analysis of neuroradiological findings showed an aqueductal stenosis, but the cause of the asymmetry was not clear.

Treatment and Outcome

At operation, the shunt was explanted and septostomy and ETV were performed. The target point for septostomy was easily found by ENS navigation (Figs. 3.33–3.36). The subarachnoid membranes were opaque and thickened. The pathway for the CSF was created through several membranes before the foramen magnum was reached (Figs. 3.37–3.41).

The postoperative course was uneventful, and MR showed a strong CSF flow (Fig. 3.42–3.45. The patient went home on the 9th day after her operation.

Fig. 3.32. This child was found on the axial MR to have an asymmetrical ventricular system (1, 2) with deviation of the pellucid septum (←). Part of a shunt system is also seen (4). The planned route for ETV and septostomy was transfrontal-transcallosal (3). The lateral aspect of MR shows a normal third ventricle and some irregularities of the foramen of Monro (↑). The aqueduct (↓) is not clearly visible. The lateral ventricle (1) is slightly hydrocephalic

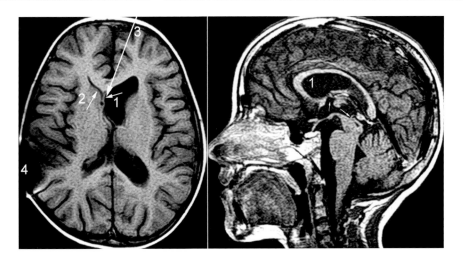

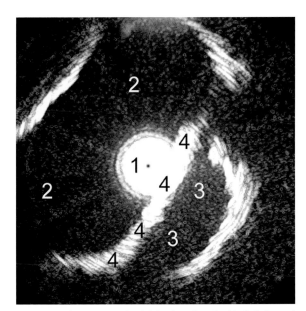

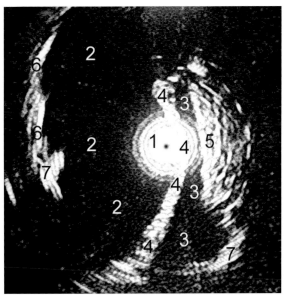

Fig. 3.33. The sono-probe (1) is placed in the big left frontal horn (2) in contact with pellucid septum (4) searching for the right perforation target to make access into the small left frontal horn (3) possible and create a communication

Fig. 3.34. The sono-probe (1) starts the perforation from the left frontal horn (2) through the pellucid septum (4) into the right frontal horn (3). The septum is bent, almost touching the lateral wall (5) of the right ventricle (3). The lateral wall (6) of the left ventricle (2) and choroid plexus (7) on both sides are visible

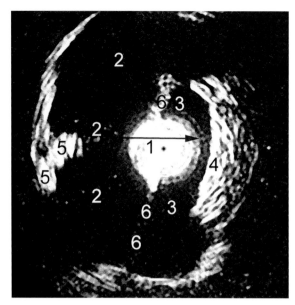

Fig. 3.35. The sono-probe (*1*) is just passing through (→) the septum (*6*) to create a communication between the left (*2*) and right (*3*) ventricles. The right (*4*) lateral ventricle wall and left choroid plexus (*5*) are shown

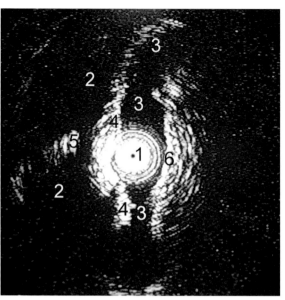

Fig. 3.36. The sono-probe (*1*) has passed from the left ventricle (*2*) through the septum (*4*) and is now in the contralateral ventricle (*3*). The small right ventricle is now enlarged by irrigation, and the right lateral wall and left plexus (*5*) are also visible

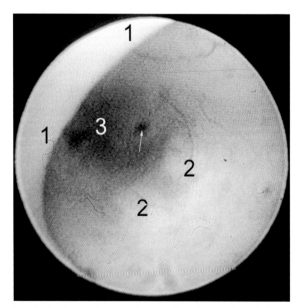

Fig. 3.37. The endoscope is introduced into the left foramen of Monro marked by the fornix (*1*). The floor of the third ventricle shows inflammatory changes, while the typical appearance is hardly recognizable. Mamillary bodies (*2*) and the infundibular recess (*3*) are barely apparent. The *dark spot* (↑) is an artifact of the lens

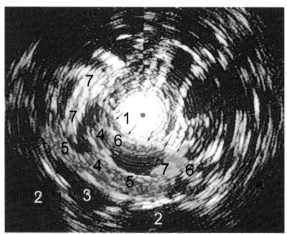

Fig. 3.38. The sono-probe (*1*) in the epiarachnoidal space is pushing the arachnoidea (↓) against the basilar head with the basilar artery (*4*) [both P1 (*5*) and right SuCA (*6*)]. The oculomotor nerves on both sides (*7*) and the interpeduncular fossa (*3*) with its cerebral peduncle (*2*) are visible

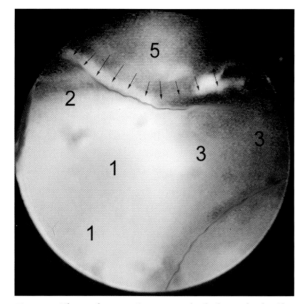

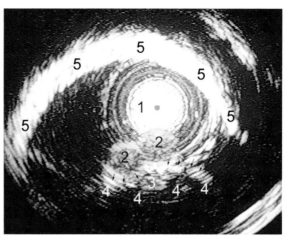

Fig. 3.39. The endoscope is now pushed along the basilar artery (*1*) inside the prepontine cistern up to the vertebrobasilar junction. The sono-probe (*5*) is pushed along an epiarachnoidal course, so that it is covered by the arachnoid membrane (↓) and positioned between the left (*2*) and the right (*3*) vertebral artery

Fig. 3.40. The sono-probe (*1*) is placed at the vertebrobasilar junction, where both vertebral arteries are just branching (*2*). The median pontine vein (*3*) is hardly visible, running in the median pontine sulcus of the pons (*4*/↓). The clivus (*5*) is visible at the level of its inner mold

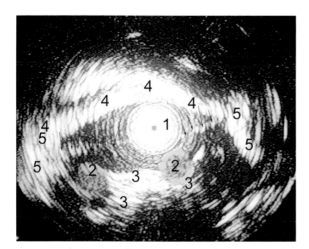

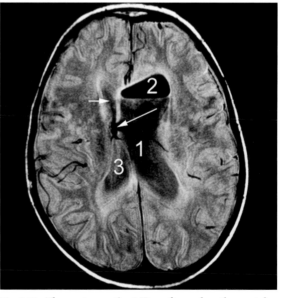

Fig. 3.41. The sono-probe (*1*) is positioned epiarachnoidally (↓) at the superior margin of the atlas (*4*). Occipital condyles (*5*) are scanned on both sides. Both vertebral arteries (*2*) are divided to the lateral sides of the medulla (*3*)

Fig. 3.42. The postoperative MR performed on the next day shows the flow of the septostomy (←) coming from the left lateral ventricle (*1*). The right lateral ventricle (*3*) is larger than preoperatively, and the frontal horn (→) is easily visible again. However, the deviation of the septum is still present and there are marked differences in the size of the lateral ventricles

3

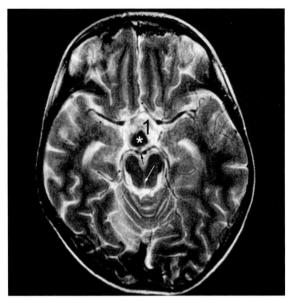

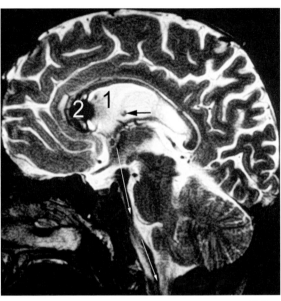

Fig. 3.43. The postoperative axial MR shows a strong flow signal (*) in the interpeduncular cistern (1) ventral to the basilar artery (↑). The aqueduct is not clearly visible in the mesencephalon (↓)

Fig. 3.44. The sagittal postoperative MR shows a small flow (←) through the septostomy and some air (2) in the lateral ventricle (1). There is a strong flow signal ventral to the brain stem (↓) into the foramen magnum

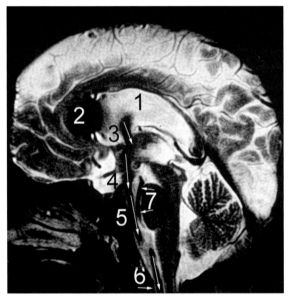

Fig. 3.45. Another phase of postoperative sagittal MR shows air (2) in the lateral ventricle (1). There are strong flow signals (↓) through the foramen of Monro (3), ventriculocisternostomy (4), along the brain stem (5) and basilar artery (7), and into the foramen magnum (6)

Case 6

Clinical History

This 16-year-old male youth was admitted to the department because of shunt nephritis. Several abdominal complications had been encountered in the past, and he had finally received a cardiac shunt. The cause of hydrocephalus was a congenital toxoplasmosis. Because of the acute shunt nephritis all shunt material had to be explanted. An X-ray of the skull and an MR investigation showed that his brain had become a 'cemetery' for old shunt catheters (Fig. 3.46, 3.47).

Complete analysis of all neuroradiological images showed an aqueductal stenosis, which is not uncommon in patients with a history of toxoplasmosis.

Treatment and Outcome

During the operation, in a first step the three blind catheters were explanted with endoscopic control (Fig. 3.48). The shunt system was then explanted and an ETV was performed (Fig. 3.49–3.53). The anatomy of the foramen of Monro and of the third ventricle floor was very much altered and was hardly recognizable in the endoscope (Fig. 3.49, 3.51). The ENS image was quite typical in appearance (Fig. 3.50, 3.52), and the first perforation during the ETV was initially done with the ENS catheter itself. Interestingly, there were no changes to the anatomy of the subarachnoidal cisterns; they also showed no signs of infection (Fig. 3.53).

The postoperative course was uneventful, so that the patient quickly recovered from his nephritis.

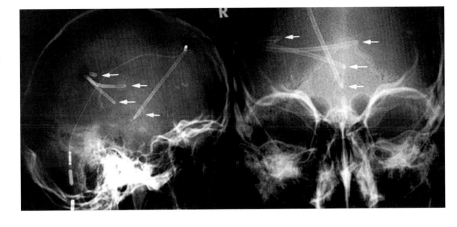

Fig. 3.46. This is a typical image of long-standing hydrocephalus and four catheters (←) in the brain. Earlier operations had shown strong adhesions between the catheters and the plexus, and they were therefore left in place

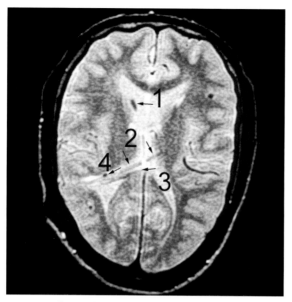

Fig. 3.47. The axial MR reveals all four catheters (1–4) and their positions relative to the brain and the ventricles

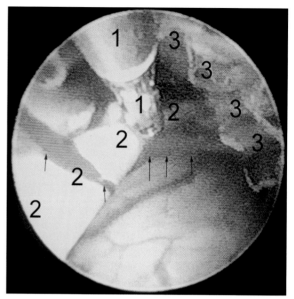

Fig. 3.48. Under endoscopic control a ventricular catheter (2) is detached with a forceps (1) from the choroid plexus (3) of the right trigone area (glomus of choroid plexus). Only minimal bleeding (↑) resulted

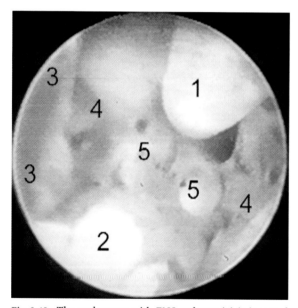

Fig. 3.49. The endoscope with ENS catheter (1) is inserted into the right foramen of Monro. The ventricular system is completely changed by inflammatory remnants, as is the foramen and some residuum of the plexus (2), while the fornix (3) is recognizable. The whole aspect of the third ventricle is changed, causing difficulties in orientation. The hypothalamus (4) and mamillary bodies (5) are hardly identifiable on either side

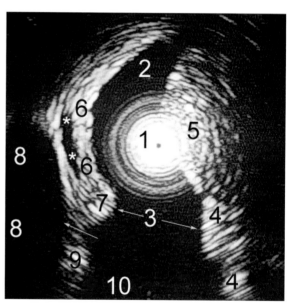

Fig. 3.50. The sono-view shows many landmarks that were altered but still helpful in orientation, being close enough to their typical shapes. The sono-probe (1) inside the frontal horn (2), still close to the caudate nucleus (5), is just in the process of becoming an enlarged foramen of Monro (3). The choroid plexus of the right lateral ventricle (4) and of the left lateral ventricle (9), also marking the left foramen of Monro (←), are seen. The pellucid septum (6) has a normal cavum (*), showing that the septum is normally double. Left frontal horn (8) and superoanterior third ventricle (10) are seen in the scan

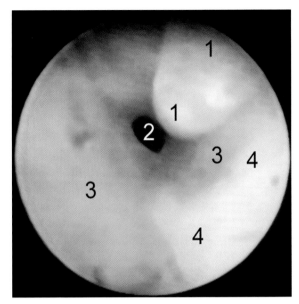

Fig. 3.51. Under endoscopic control, the sono-probe (1) is used to create the primary perforation (2), presenting parallel real-time and online sono-monitoring (navigation) (see Fig. 3.52). Mamillary bodies (3) are hardly visible, the view being hampered by the choroid plexus (4) of the foramen of Monro

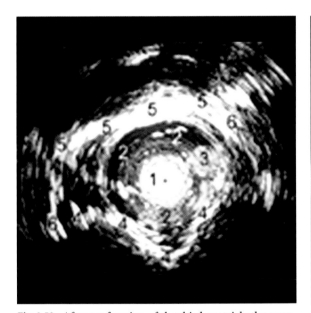

Fig. 3.52. After perforation of the third ventricle the sono-probe (1) 'sees' what the endoscope does not see: the clearest landmark signal of the sellar dorsum (5), the typical peduncular shape of the ventral mesencephalon (4), the interpeduncular fossa (2), and basilar artery (3). On the monitor all pulsations, flows, and movements of arachnoid membranes (↑), and also the sono-probe itself (1) are visible in real time. Laterally on both sides the tentorial notch (6) is seen

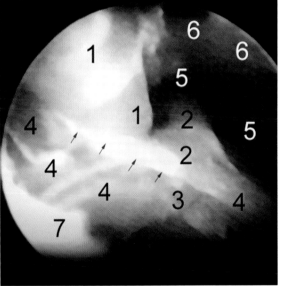

Fig. 3.53. The endoscope has followed the sono-probe (1), finding it lateral to the basilar artery (2) on the left, as expected from the sono-scan image (Fig. 3.52). The basilar bifurcation (3) into the two P1 segments (1) is visible, as is some arachnoid tissue. The light gets lost in the depth of the prepontine cistern (5) and clivus (6)

Cystic Lesions

Cystic lesions (Table 3.3) are always ideal candidates for endoscopy: in cases of multiple cysts, intra-parenchymal cyst walls, and narrow and complex borders of lesions, the sono-catheter can give additional information and enhance the safety level by providing intraoperative imaging and supporting the navigation.

In the case of a *velum interpositum cyst*, orientation, precise navigation, and targeting of the perforation point combine to pose a high-risk problem. In such specific cases in this series the communication could not be maintained by means of the endoscope only. Additionally, in one case a bleed meant that the procedure could not be successfully finished except with the aid of the second image of the sono-scan, because with impaired vision the risk was too high.

Arachnoid cysts, for example at the temporal base, need a communication to be made into the tentorial slit. There is a risk of injuring the ICA, the PcoA, and the oculomotor nerve. With the sono-catheter, however, it is possible to target the recommended perforation area precisely. Navigation is possible independently of ventricular changes or shifting because of the real-time imaging with ENS.

One of the indications for which use of ENS proved most impressive was *multicystic hydrocephalus*. In these cases the main problem was navigation. Most of the patients were children who had had unacceptably high numbers of operations. The objective was to make them shunt free, especially when abdominal scarification, shunt nephritis, multiple shunt failures, or shunt infections were present. In these cases complex stomas and perforations were needed, which were riskier than frequent endoscopic procedures. The sono-scan guided the endoscope in phases in which visual problems arose, allowing precise and safe navigation of the endoscope to the site targeted for perforation.

Table 3.3. Cystic lesions

Type of cystic lesion	n
Arachnoid cyst (1 case + aneurysm)	2
Velum interpositum cyst	1
Colloid cyst	2
Sellar cyst	1
Pinealis	1
Abscess	1
Ventricle	2

Case 7

Clinical History

This 56-year-old woman was admitted after an attack with speech arrest and hypesthesia of the hands during a stressful situation. The MR showed a double cyst close to the right lateral ventricle and a slight shift of the midline (Figs. 3.54).

Treatment and Outcome

An operation was done transendoscopically with ENS navigation. The two cysts were connected, and a fenestration into the lateral ventricle was performed (Fig. 3.55, 3.56). Intraoperative histology showed that an astrocytoma grade I was present. The biopsy area showed a higher echo density than the brain tissue on sono-imaging (Fig. 3.57). This area was then resected endoscopically.

The postoperative course was uneventful, and the patient went home on the 10th day after surgery.

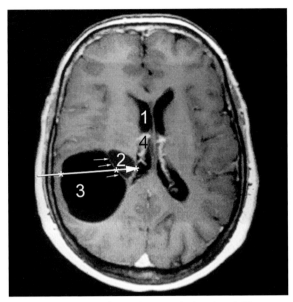

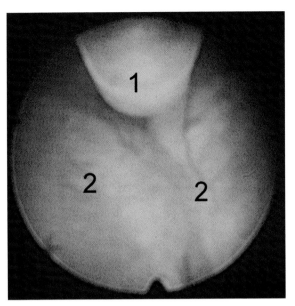

Fig. 3.54. This MR of a multicystic lesion (2, 3) illustrates the neuronavigation problem of how to find the perforation targets (*). A communication route (→) must be found to drain both cysts into the lateral ventricle (1)

Fig. 3.55. Endoscopic view into the large cyst (2) (see *part 3*) shows the sono-probe (1) and the typical appearance of such cysts, having no landmarks at all for orientation

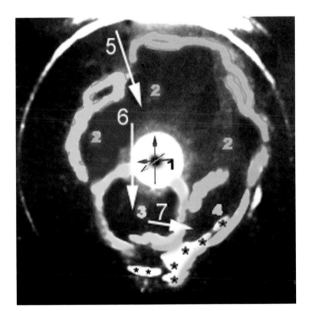

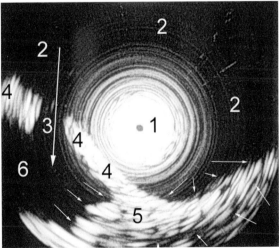

Fig. 3.56. The sono-probe (1) is seen in the real-time imaging and can be navigated (↑←↓→) inside the large cyst (2) to the small cyst (3) and into the lateral ventricle (4). Three perforations (↓) have been made: one into the large cyst (5), one into the small cyst (6), and one into the ventricle (7), which was easily recognizable from the strong echo signals of the choroid plexus (***)

Fig. 3.57. The sono-probe (1) inside the large cyst (2) showed the perforation (3) of the membrane (4) into the small cyst (6) and a hyperechogenic zone (→5←), which proved to be an astrocytoma I on histology

Case 8

Clinical History

This 2-year-old girl presented with a change in behavior that had started 2 weeks before her admission. A cyst in the velum interpositum had been detected on sonographic examination when the girl was 6 months old.

MR showed the dimensions of the cyst precisely (Fig. 3.58–3.60): it was pushing the roof of the third ventricle downward and forward. There were several possible trajectories for creating a communication between the cyst and the ventricles (Fig. 3.61, 3.62).

Treatment and Outcome

The route from the ventricular trigone into the cyst was finally chosen (Fig. 3.63, 3.64). The postoperative MR showed a broad communication and a reduction in size, as well as release of compression on the neighboring structures.

The girl left hospital on the 8th postoperative day, presenting a normal neurological and clinical condition.

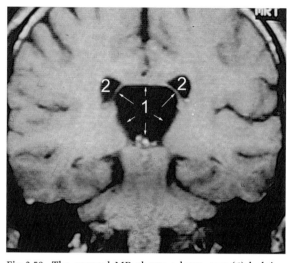

Fig. 3.58. The coronal MR shows a large cyst (*1*) bulging (→) into the third ventricle and even toward the lateral ventricles (*2*)

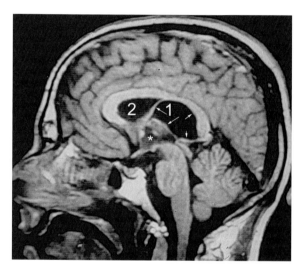

Fig. 3.59. In the lateral MR it becomes obvious that the cyst (*1*) is in the velum interpositum (telo-diencephalic fissure), compressing (→) the third ventricle (*) and the lateral ventricle (*2*)

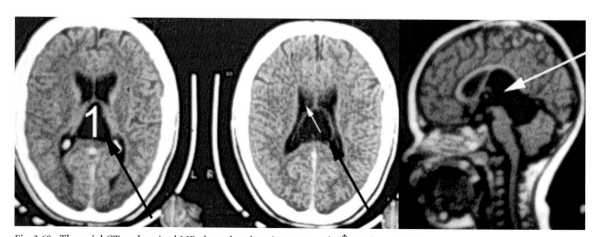

Fig. 3.60. The axial CT and sagittal MR show the planning approach (↑) to the cyst (*1*)

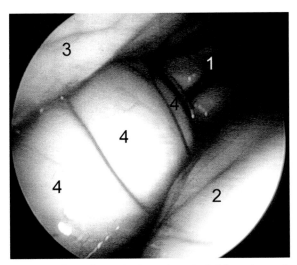

Fig. 3.61. The endoscopic view is into the left lateral ventricle (1) from occipital. Between the lateral (2) and medial (3) walls there is the bulging cyst (4)

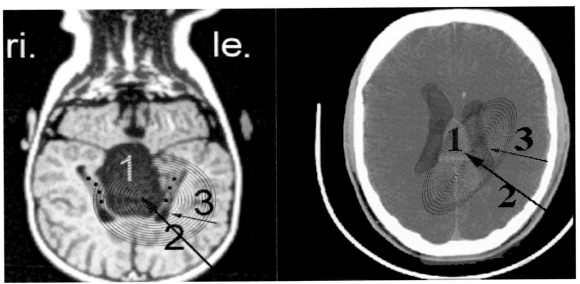

Fig. 3.62. This coronal upside-down MR shows the planning as seen by the surgeon during the operation. The route (2) to the cyst (1) runs through the left lateral ventricle (3) superior to the choroid plexus (...)

3

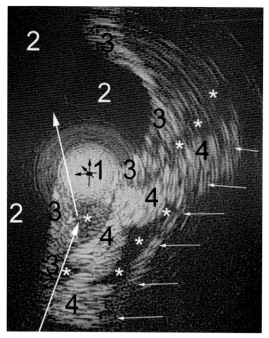

Fig. 3.63. The sono-probe (*1*) is just perforating (↑ the lateral ventricle (*) with the choroid plexus (*4*) through the wall (*3*) of the cyst (*2*). The lateral wall (←) of the ventricle (*) is close to the cyst, as it is compressed

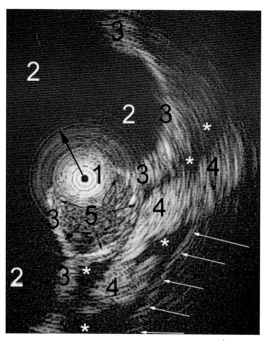

Fig. 3.64. The sono-probe (*1*) is perforating (↑) the membrane (*3*) of the cyst (*2*), causing a small hemorrhage (*5*) into the cavity (←→) between the wall (*3*) of the cyst (*2*) and the lateral ventricle (*). The choroid plexus as landmark of the ventricle (*4*) and the lateral wall (←) of the ventricle are easily visible

Colloid Cyst

Ventricular tumors frequently present as cysts on MRI or CT. In all our cases the sono-catheter correctly predicted the difference between cyst and tumor. In patients with *colloid cysts* it was possible to predict the viscosity of the content. It was helpful to know this before the puncture was made. Larger vessels, cystic areas, different consistencies of the tumor, and the border with the parenchyma were visible on the scan before penetration.

Case 9

Clinical History

This 25-year-old man had a long history of headache attacks. He reported worsening concentration and difficulties in remembering new information. MR showed the typical finding of a colloid cyst (Fig. 3.65).

The ENS image predicted the consistency of the cyst material and its attachment to endoscopically invisible vessels (Fig. 3.66–3.68).

Treatment and Outcome

Because of strong adhesions, the cyst was removed microsurgically and endoscopic control subsequently confirmed complete resection.

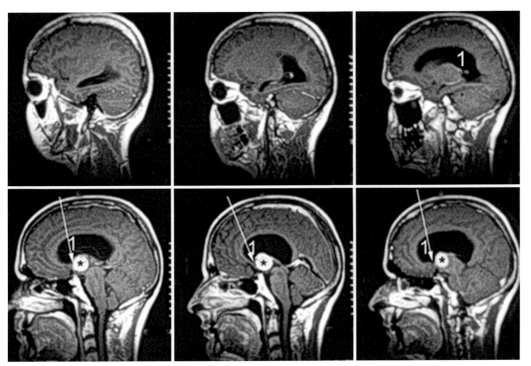

Fig. 3.65. The sagittal MR showed the typical appearance of a colloid cyst (*) with hydrocephalus of lateral ventricles (*1*). Moreover, a consecutive occlusive hydrocephalus was present. A transfrontal-transventricular approach (↓) was planned

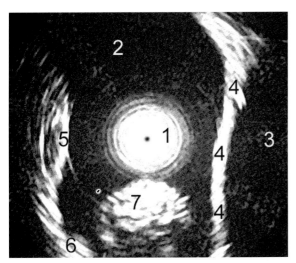

Fig. 3.66. The sono-probe (*1*) is in the left frontal horn (*2*) scanning the right frontal horn (*3*) through the pellucid septum (*4*). It is in contact with the colloid cyst (*7*) and depicts choroid plexus (*6*) and caudate nucleus (*5*)

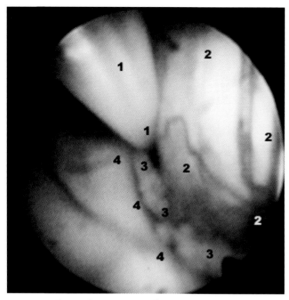

Fig. 3.67. The endoscope sees the sono-catheter (*1*) entering the foramen of Monro (↓) in contact with the colloid cyst (*2*), the choroid plexus (*3*) and the fornix (*4*)

Tumors

Tumors (Table 3.4) are very different in their echo signal, which is helpful in their detection and their differentiation from normal tissue or CSF. Meningiomas, craniopharyngiomas, colloid cysts, and acoustic neurinomas are well delineated by the sonoprobe. Hypophyseal tumors and astrocytomas are not well differentiated from normal tissue. However, borders to the CSF and to the bone could always be well defined. The main problems in resection monitoring were the well-known changes of resection planes. However, a craniopharyngioma remnant hidden by the optic nerve and not even seen by the endoscope was well detected. Two microadenomas of the pituitary gland and one metastasis in a pituitary adenoma were hardly visible, however. On the other hand, the borders of hypophyseal tumors could be well demonstrated on the CSF and cavernous sinus side. Contact with the ICA was easily recognized by the blood flow. The sonographic image resolution was high, even at such deep levels, because the sonoprobe could always be positioned directly on the target in deep narrow spaces.

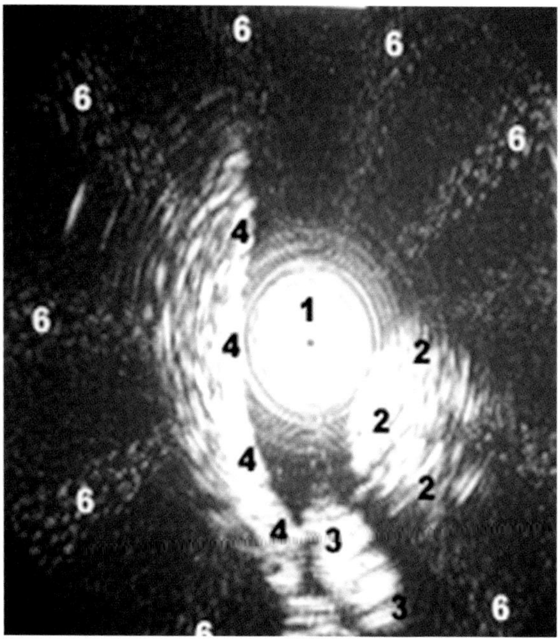

Fig. 3.68. The sono-probe (*1*) view correlates exactly with the endoscopic view in Fig. 3.67, and it is in contact with the colloid cyst (*2*) close to the choroid plexus (*3*) and to the fornix (*4*). The pellucid septum (*5*) and a rotation artifact (*6*) are also visible

Table 3.4. Tumor cases

Tumor type	*n*
Hemangioblastoma (cerebellar)	1
Craniopharygioma	1
Meningioma (tubercle of sella turcica, cerebellopontine)	2
Colloid cyst	2
Epidermoid (orbita)	1
Acoustic neurinoma	2
Astrocytoma	7
Hypophyseal tumor	6

Case 10

This 29-year-old man presented with a 6-week history of intermittent hypesthesia of the right side of the face followed by weakness of the right leg, lasting for some minutes each time. Neurological findings were normal.

MR showed a tumor in the posterior third ventricle with aqueduct compression and three-ventricular hydrocephalus.

Endoscopic inspection (Fig. 3.69) gave the impression of tissue and compression of neighboring structures. A biopsy specimen was examined, and the diagnosis was benign astrocytoma. ENS imaging (Fig. 3.70, 3.71) showed clear delineation of tumor borders not only in the third ventricle but also in the thalamic tissue. The final histological diagnosis was pilocytic astrocytoma WHO I.

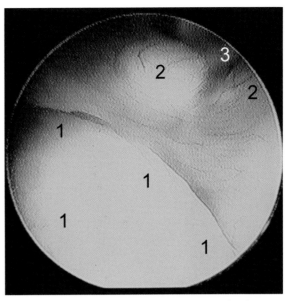

Fig. 3.69. The endoscope is now placed in the third ventricle, where part of a glioma (1) is visible. Mamillary bodies (2) and membranous infundibulum (3) can be used as landmarks

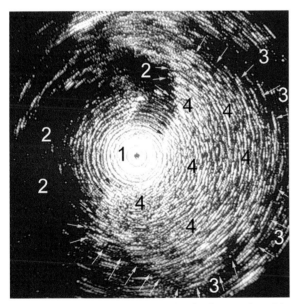

Fig. 3.70. The sono-probe (1) is in the third ventricle and in contact with the tumor (4). The borders of the tumor (→←) are visible on the same side as the ventricle (2) and, interestingly, also towards the same side as the thalamus (3)

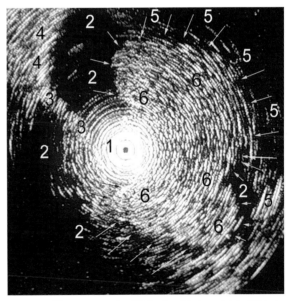

Fig. 3.71. The sono-probe (1) in the third ventricle (2) is in contact with the hydrocephalic stretched interthalamic adhesion (3) and with the tumor (6). The border of the tumor (→←) is well delineated toward the third ventricle (2), but also toward the normal tissue of the thalamus (5). The left thalamus is also visible

3

Sellar Region

Case 11

Clinical History
This 41-year-old man complained of deficiency in the visual field and had some signs of diabetes insipidus. MR showed a cystic craniopharyngioma of the pituitary stalk, which was compressing the floor of the third ventricle.

Treatment and Outcome
Intraoperatively, ENS was used for resection control. Targeting for remnants invisible to the microscope or to the endoscope was achieved with a picture-in-picture (PIP) technique (Figs. 3.72, 3.73).

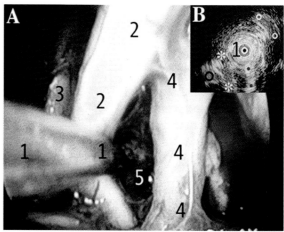

Figs. 3.72, 3.73. This view seen by the surgeon in a PIP presentation through the HMD system includes an endoscopic view (*A*) and the sono-scan (*B*), both in real time and online in parallel. The sono-probe (*A+B1*) is positioned between the right optic nerve (*2*) and the right carotid artery (*4*) in the retrosellar area (*5*). In the field that is not visible, the sonographic view (*B*) represents the left infra-clinoidal carotid artery (* *) and the right carotid artery (° °) and also a remnant of a calcified craniopharyngioma (. .). The left optic nerve is visible in both the endoscope (*A3*) and the ENS view (*B* °)

Case 12

Clinical History

This 67-year-old lady had had prior laser therapy because of retinal bleeding 6 years before admission. Five years before CT findings had been normal, and MR examination 2 years previously had shown the sellar cyst, but the patient had refused surgery. Finally her vision deteriorated and she experienced hypopituitarism.

Treatment and Outcome

Preoperative CT showed a large sellar cyst (Fig. 3.74, 1), and MR confirmed the compression of optic chiasm (Fig. 74, 2, 3). An operation was done with the PIP technique, and ENS confirmed the presence of a residual fragment of the pituitary gland (Figs. 3.75–3.78).

Fig. 3.74. Axial CT shows an enlarged sella (1). The coronal MR shows compression of the optic chiasm attributable to a tumor or cyst (1). The sagittal MR represents the sella with a high signal (2)

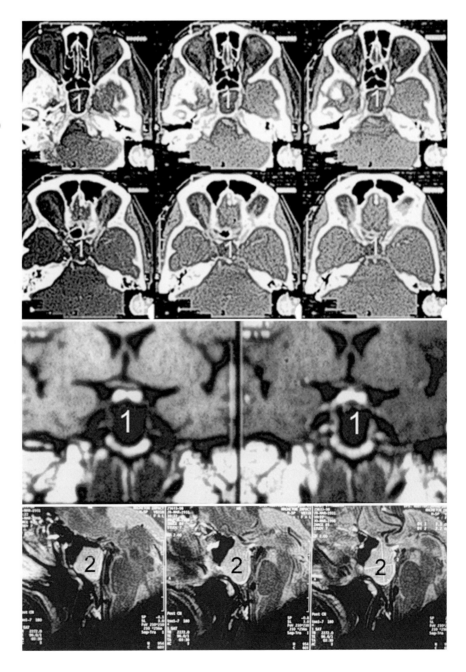

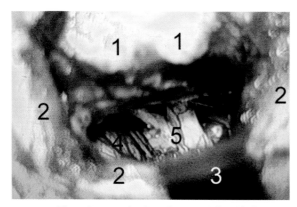

Fig. 3.75. The microscopic view shows a right-sided supra-orbital approach with orbital rim (1), soft tissue, and skin (2). A 1-cm spatula (3) is lifting the frontal lobe (4) and allowing sight of the optic chiasm with both optic nerves (5)

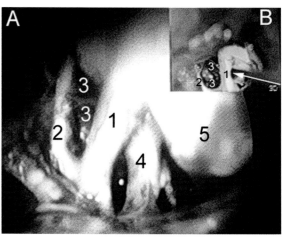

Fig. 3.76A, B. In the PIP presentation of an endoscopic view (A) and the microscopic view (B) monitoring the endoscope (←) we see the right (1) and left (2) optic nerves and an enlarged sella (3) within an arachnoid cyst

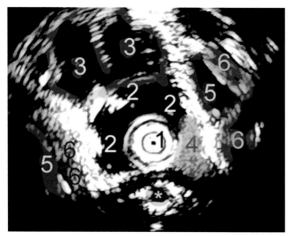

Fig. 3.77. The sono-probe (1) is in the sellar cyst (2), detecting a rest of the pituitary gland (4). The cranial rest of the sphenoid sinus with a septum is visible (3), and lateral to the sella the cavernous sinus (5) is seen within the carotid artery (6) on both sides. A strongly calcified basilar artery (*) close to the clivus is scanned

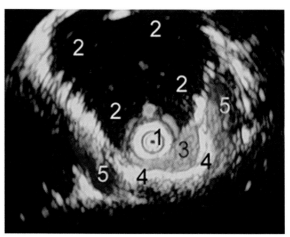

Fig. 3.78. The sono-probe (1) is placed into the sellar cyst (2) in contact with a rest of the pituitary gland (3) deep in the clivus (4). Inside the cavernous sinus the carotid artery (5) is visible on both sides

Case 13

Clinical History

This 50-year-old man was admitted with bitemporal hemianopsia and ataxia on walking. MR showed a meningioma of the sellar tubercle, and also depicted obstructive hydrocephalus caused by aqueductal stenosis (Figs. 3.79, 3.80). The hormonal function of the somatotropic axis was impaired.

Treatment and Outcome

On operation from a right-sided pterional approach, the tumor was found to be compressing both optic nerves and the lamina terminalis was bulging. The first step was to perforate the lamina terminalis, creating a ventriculocisternostomy and releasing the pressure on both optic nerves (Fig. 3.81).

ENS imaging presented a precise anatomical relation between tumor, carotid artery, and cranial base with contacting borders invisible to the microscope (Figs. 3.82–3.84). No invasion of the carotid artery or of the sphenoid sinus was seen during inspection of the tumor bed (Fig. 3.85).

Postoperative rhinoliquorrhea was observed, which was successfully treated by several days of lumbar drainage. The patient left the clinic in an excellent condition on the 17th day after surgery.

Fig. 3.79. MR coronal shows the meningioma (*) of the sellar tubercle with compression (↓) of the optic chiasm and hydrocephalus (*1*) in addition

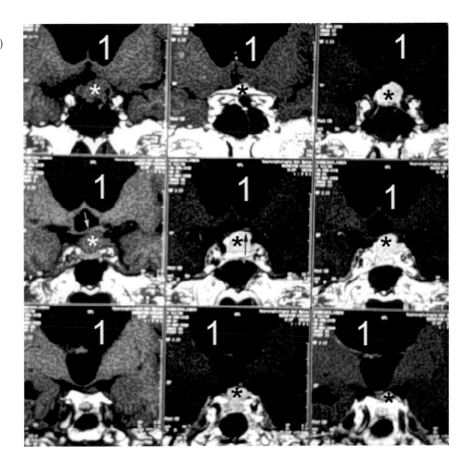

3

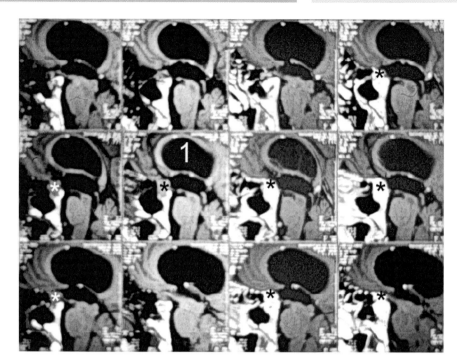

Fig. 3.80. MR sagittal shows the tumor (*) and the hydrocephalus (1) with and without gadolinium

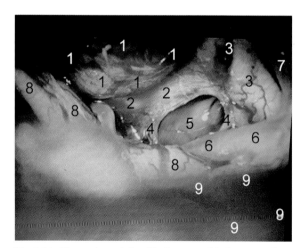

Fig. 3.81. Through a right-sided supraorbital approach, a meningioma (1) of the tubercle of the sella is visible, compressing the optic chiasm (2). The lamina terminalis (4) is opened for release of more CSF, and the anterior third ventricle (5) is open. The right optic nerve (3) and right carotid artery (7) and branching A1 (6) are approached. A spatula (9) is placed under the frontal lobe (8)

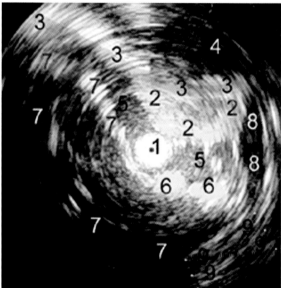

Fig. 3.82. The sono-probe (1) is placed in the suprasellar subarachnoid space (5) in contact with the meningioma (2) on the tubercle (3) of the sella, part of which is the roof of the sphenoid sinus (4). The CSF (5) is not clear, and there are two artifacts caused by blood-soaked pads (6). The frontal lobe (7) is lifted with a spatula, which is seen as a typical spatula artifact (...9...). The meningioma (2) can be seen to be in contact with the right infraclinoidal ICA (8)

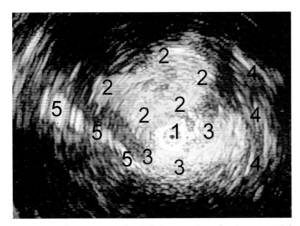

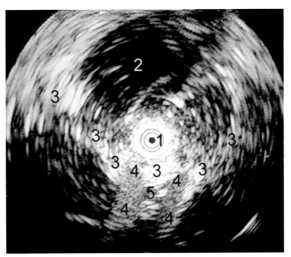

Fig. 3.83. The sono-probe (*1*) is entering the intracranial space between the meningioma (*2*) and the optic chiasm (*3*), which is hardly visible, and the lateral right ICA (*4*). The basal surface of the frontal lobe (*5*) gives a strong signal

Fig. 3.84. The sono-probe (*1*) is placed subfrontally (*2*) in the midline and close to the frontal lobe (*3*). Coincidentally, both A1 entering A2 (*4*) and CoA (*5*) are in the scan plane

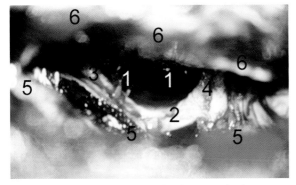

Fig. 3.85. Through the supraorbital approach the tumor bed (*1*) after resection is visible, as are the optic chiasm (*2*) left (*3*) and right (*4*) and the optic nerves. The field of vision is limited by the frontal lobe (*5*) and orbital rim (*6*)

3

Transnasal Approach to Sellar Region

The transnasal approach is ideal for imaging by ENS, as it leaves only a small gap for working. The imaging geometry results in frontal scans of the region (Figs. 3.86–3.89).

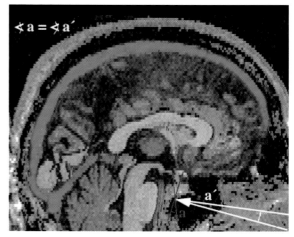

Fig. 3.86. The ENS catheter (*white* ←) can be inserted transnasally and will then give a coronal image (*red* ↔) of the sellar region. The angle of the ENS catheter will be reflected in the angle of the coronal imaging plane

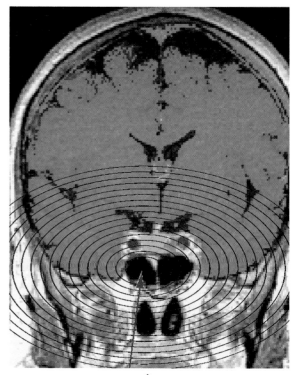

Fig. 3.87. The ENS catheter (↑) will produce a frontal plane image of the sellar region. The angle of the plane depends on the angle of the catheter direction

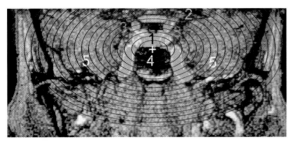

Fig. 3.88. With the patient in the half-sitting position and face to face with the surgeon, the transnasal ENS shows a frontal plane image. The sono-catheter (+) is placed in the sphenoid sinus (4), and the sella with the pituitary gland (1), the carotid artery (3) with several cuts, and the optic chiasm (2) can be seen within the scan

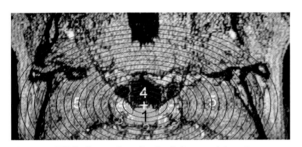

Fig. 3.89. With the patient in the lying position the transnasal ENS shows an upside-down frontal plane image. The sono-catheter (+) is placed in the sphenoid sinus (4) and sella with the pituitary gland (1), while the optic nerves (2) are seen below the catheter. Laterally, on both sides the carotid artery (3) is hardly visible in any of several cuts. The temporal lobe is outside of the imaging scope

Case 14

Clinical History

This 70-year-old patient underwent MR examination because of Parkinson's disease, and an intrasellar tumor was found on this occasion. There was no hormonal hyperactivity, and no hypophyseal deficit was found on edocrinological examination.

Treatment and Outcome

On MR, the tumor was seen to be perforating the sellar floor (Fig. 3.90) and ENS imaging showed a good correlation with preoperative MR (Fig. 3.91). The tumor was seen to reach the cavernous sinus on MR, which also showed good correlation with ENS (Fig. 3.92).

Postoperatively the patient did well, and hormonal replacement therapy was not necessary.

Case 15

This 55-year-old woman had had an operation to remove a hypopharyngeal carcinoma 15 months before her admission. At the control examination and after radiation she presented with abducens paresis on the left and accessorius and hypoglossal paresis and hemihypesthesia on the right, all of which were new symptoms after radiation.

Neuroradiological examination showed a large sella and an intra- and suprasellar tumor (Fig. 3.93–3.96). The 3D system used to plan the operation approach shows the direction of the ENS catheter (Fig. 3.97), which was used freehand in this case.

ENS imaging showed an atypical appearance of sellar tumor (Fig. 3.98), which was quite inhomogeneous. Intraoperative histology made it possible to diagnose a metastasis of a carcinoma.

3

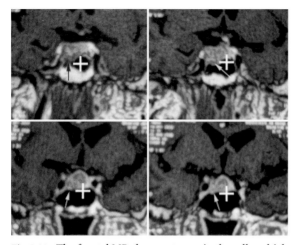

Fig. 3.90. The frontal MR shows a tumor in the sella, which broke through the sella floor (↑) into the sphenoid sinus, where the sono-probe (+) is placed

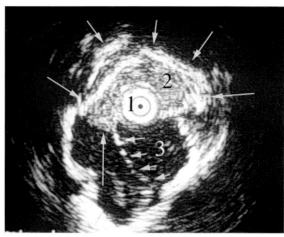

Fig. 3.91. The sono-probe (1) is in the sphenoid sinus (3), touching the dura of the sellar floor and showing the pituitary gland (2), with the tumor (↑) protruding into the sphenoid sinus. The bony wall of the anterior sella (↓) and a septum (←) of the sphenoid sinus are visible

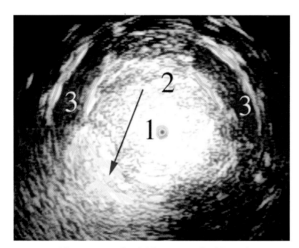

Fig. 3.92. The sono-probe (1) is now pushed into the tumor (2). The protruding part of the tumor (↓) is clearly visible. Lateral to the sella, both carotid arteries (3) are scanned

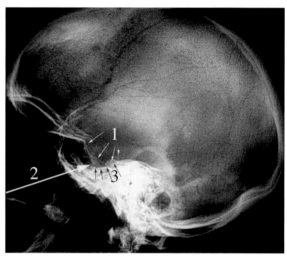

Fig. 3.93. This is the typical appearance of an enlarged sella (1/↓), seen laterally. The ENS catheter (2) is introduced transnasally (→). To get beneath the sella, the subsellar bone of the clivus (3/↑) had to be drilled to create enough space for the catheter. This can be planned according to individual neuroradiological findings

Fig. 3.94. Sagittal MR shows a sellar tumor (*) with a suprasellar part (→)

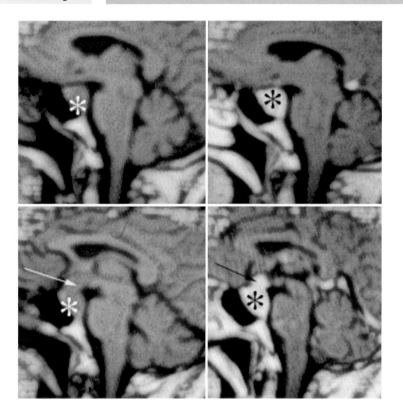

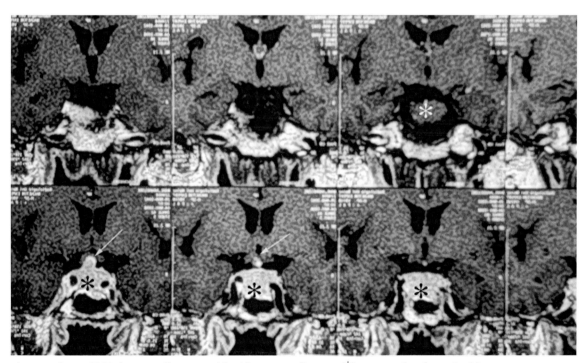

Fig. 3.95. Coronal MR shows a sellar tumor (*) with a suprasellar part (↓) compressing the optic chiasm

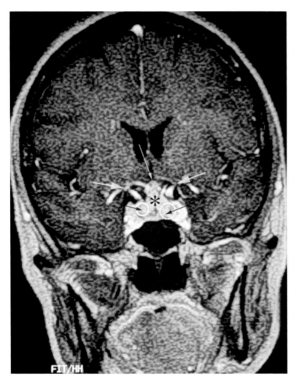

Fig. 3.96. The coronal MR shows an inhomogeneous tumor (*) with enhancement in different parts (→O←) and a suprasellar part (↓) compressing the optic chiasm and in contact with the ICA bifurcation (⇒⇐) on both sides

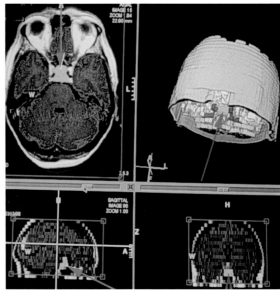

Fig. 3.97. A 3D planning system shows the position of the ENS catheter (*red arrow*). Such non-real-time images may help to make interpretation of ENS images easier and give the main orientation

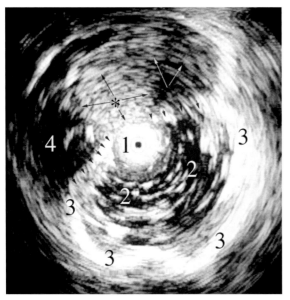

Fig. 3.98. The sono-probe (*1*) is placed in the sphenoid sinus (*2*) with a strong bony wall (*3*) and is in contact with the sellar dura (↓↓). Inside the sella (*4*) there are a tumor (*) and several inhomogeneous enhancements (↑). Histology allowed diagnosis of a metastasis of a carcinoma

Posterior Fossa

Case 16

Clinical History

This 49-year-old patient had experienced left ana-cousis 2 years before her operation in our clinic. After rheological therapy her hearing was restored. One year later she had a second anacousis attack followed by urgent diagnostic MR. An intracisternal acoustic neurinoma was found; her hearing was minimal, and acoustically evoked potentials (AEPS) were diminished.

Intraoperative viewing (Fig. 3.99) showed a spherical tumor, reaching from tentorium to jugular foramen. ENS imaging (Fig. 3.100–3.102) presented a clear delineation of the tumor borders and of most surrounding structures. However, it was not possible to see the facial nerve attached to the tu-mor. Petrosal structures and sinuses were visible, and the meatus was filled completely by the tumor. Intraoperative real-time imaging showed details invisible to conventional ultrasound probes in the deep tissue.

Treatment and Outcome

Tumor resection was achieved by microsurgery with endoscopic resection control, especially in the meatus. Facial function was intact postoperatively, and the patient's hearing had recovered some-what.

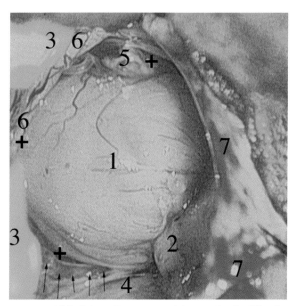

Fig. 3.99. This large CPA tumor (1) completely fills the meatus of the petrosal bone (2) and almost reaches the ten-torium (4), where it touches a small vein (↑) close to the ambient cistern. The caudal margin reaches the lateral cerebellomedullary cistern (5). Two spatulas (3) are pro-tecting the cerebellum (6), and the dura (7) is reflected lat-erally. The ENS catheter is placed in three different posi-tions (+)

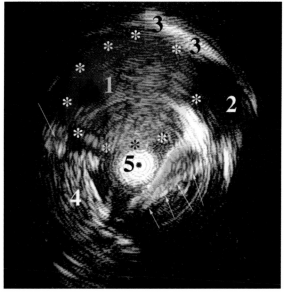

Fig. 3.100. The sono-probe (5) is placed between the supe-rior border of the tumor (1) and a small petrosal vein (↑), in which blood flow is visible on the screen or video. The pons and a spatula artifact (4) are visible, as is a small artery, in an axial scan (↓). The border of the tumor (*) gives a round signal, attached to the petrosal bone (3) with pneumatic areas (2)

3

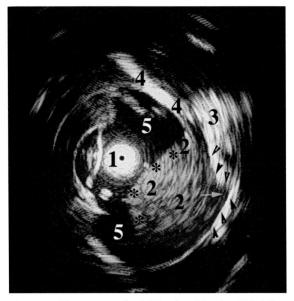

Fig. 3.101. The sono-probe (*1*) is placed in the CPA (*5*) at the tumor equator (*). The tumor (*2*) has enlarged (*arrowheads*) the meatus (*arrow*). The roof of the jugular bulb (*3*) and the clivus (*4*) are visible

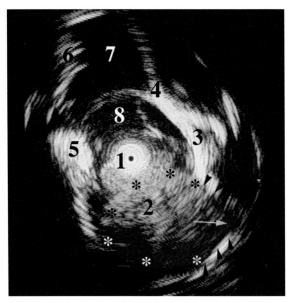

Fig. 3.102. The sono-probe (*1*) is placed in the lateral cerebellomedullary cistern (*8*) at the inferior border (*) of the tumor (*2*). The wide opening (*thick arrow*) of the meatus (→) is visible, as is the jugular bulb (*3*). On the brain side Bochdalek's bodies are present (*5*), and caudally the subarachnoid way into foramen magnum (*7*) is within the scan

Case 17

Clinical History
This 46-year-old man had had two operations for cerebellar hemangioblastoma at the age of 15 and 18 years. Now, 31 years after the first operation and 28 years after the second, he was experiencing progressive impairment of walking.

MR showed a cystic relapse of the tumor (Fig. 3.103–3.105) in the cerebellum and in the dorsal medulla oblongata.

Treatment and Outcome
Intraoperative localization was not easy, as the cyst walls did not allow observation of the tumor. ENS was used for easy real-time imaging and targeting of the tumors (Fig. 3.106–3.108). ENS was used to help check that resection was complete.

Postoperatively, the patient's symptoms started to diminish, but 1 month later he developed hydrocephalus. An ETV was planned, but the surgeon did not use ENS and was not able to perform an adequate stomy, as there was not enough space. However, a shunt was finally inserted. Up to October 2000 several revision operations had been necessary because of tumor recurrences, spinal tumors, and shunt problems.

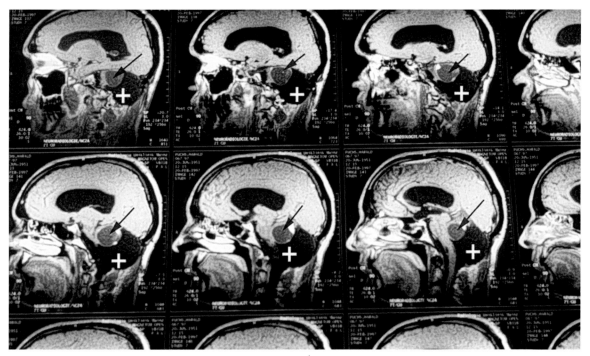

Fig. 3.103. Sagittal MR shows a recurrence of a Lindau tumor (↓) and an old resection cavity (+)

Fig. 3.104. This axial MR shows an old resection cavity (+) with a Lindau tumor (*). The tumor nodule (↑) is seen within the cyst

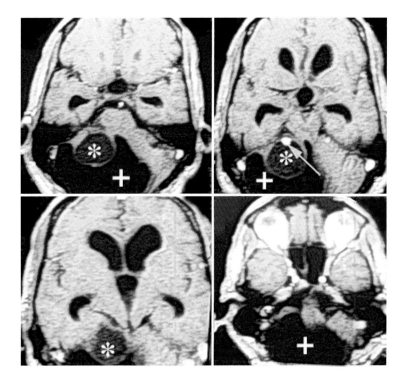

3

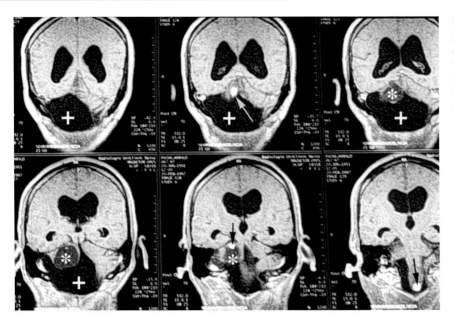

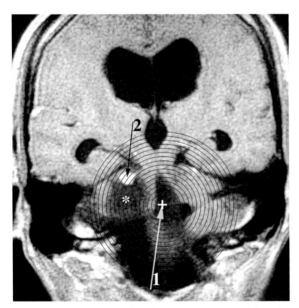

Fig. 3.106. The sono-probe (*1*), which is positioned in the fourth ventricle (+), as shown in Fig. 107, imaging a coronal plane (⊕). The tumor nodule (*2*) and tumor cyst (*) are within the scan

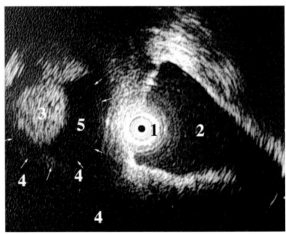

Fig. 3.107. The sono-probe (*1*) is inside the fourth ventricle (*2*), which like the tumor cyst (*5*) or the old resection cavity (*4*), was a cystic cavity. On entry into the fourth ventricle it was not at all clear which cystic space was present and where the tumor nodule (*3*) was to be found. ENS produced a precise real-time topography (see Fig. 3.106) for navigation to the Lindau tumor (*3*)

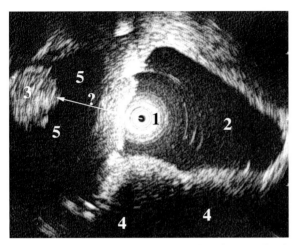

Fig. 3.108. The sono-probe (*1*) is in the fourth ventricle (*2*) and can navigate instruments or the endoscope to the Lindau tumor (*3*) with its cyst (*5*) or make a communication to the cavity (*4*)

Case 18

In this case, the approaches were planned in 3D, and the use of ENS was demonstrated virtually (Figs. 3.109–3.112).

Clinical History

This 66-year-old man had been suffering from trigeminal neuralgia for 10 years. Carbamazepine was used for primary pain control, but the dose had to be increased more and more and eventually the side effects became unacceptable. Neuroradiological examinations showed typical contact of the anterior inferior cerebellar artery (AICA) with the trigeminal nerve entry zone.

Operative planning with 3D reconstruction and computer assistance gave the impression of a method of approach design and anatomical relationships. The geometry of ENS imaging was demonstrated (Figs. 3.109–3.112).

Treatment and Outcome

At operation, ENS imaging of the lateral-suboccipital approach was demonstrable (Figs. 3.113–3.116) plus the compression point of the trigeminal nerve, which was not visible on endoscopy (Fig. 3.117).

Postoperatively, the patient did well and the trigeminal neuralgia disappeared.

3

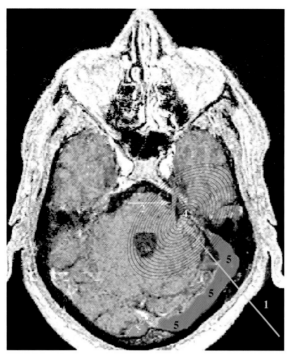

Fig. 3.109. The ENS catheter (1) was introduced by a right lateral suboccipital approach into the CPA. Under the transverse sinus (5) the trigeminal nerve (3) compressed (2) by an AICA loop (4) was approached and examined

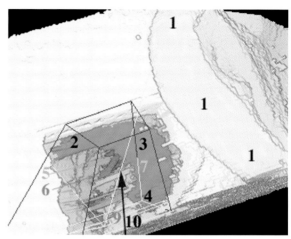

Fig. 3.110. This is a 3D representation of an operation planning-system, representing a right suboccipital approach through which the ENS catheter (10/↑) is inserted into the CPA cisterns. The computer reconstruction shows the right ear (1), transverse sinus (2), sinus knee (3) and sigmoid sinus (4). In the deep tissues the Vth (5) and VIIth/VIIIth (7) cranial nerves and the jugular nerve bundle (8) are visible. Close to the trigeminal nerve (5) there is an AICA loop (6), and close to the jugular nerve bundle the posterior inferior cerebellar artery (PICA) (9) is visible

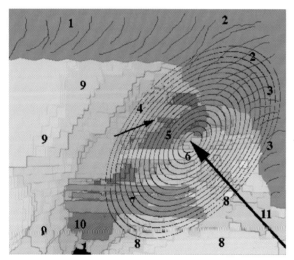

Fig. 3.111. The virtual view into the right CPA shows the position of the ENS catheter (11) producing soundwaves (()). At the laterosuperior border we see the transverse sinus (1), the sinus knee (2), and the sigmoid sinus (3). The Vth (4) and VIIth/VIIIth (6) cranial nerves and the jugular nerve bundle (7) running between brain stem (9) and petrosus bone (8) are visible. An AICA loop (5) and the PICA (10) are close to neighboring nerves

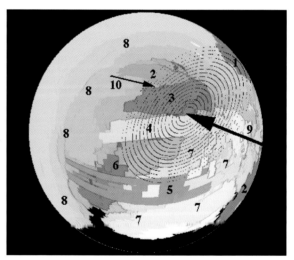

Fig. 3.112. This virtual endoscopy in the right CPA shows the position of the ENS catheter (9) with ultrasound waves (()), and CPA between brain stem (8) and petrosus bone (7). Transverse sinus (1) and sigmoid sinus are just coming into view. The trigeminal nerve (2) is close (→) to an AICA loop (3) and the 7/8 bundle (4). The jugular nerve bundle (5) is in contact with the PICA (5)

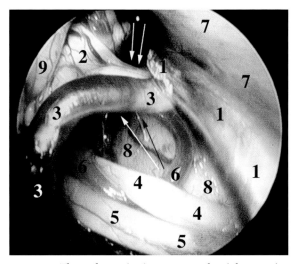

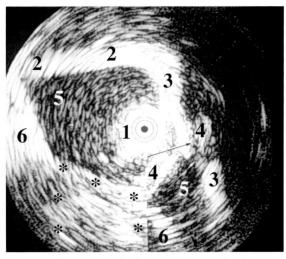

Fig. 3.113. The endoscopic view presents the right superior cerebellar artery (SUCA). The sono-probe (1) is placed superior to the trigeminal nerve (2), which together with Dandy's vein (3) runs toward the petrosal bone (8) and the tentorium (7). Between these, the facial nerve (4), the acoustic nerve (5), and the AICA loop (6) run cranially below the trigeminal nerve (↑), causing neuralgia (↓)

Fig. 3.114. The sono-probe (1) is inserted into the right CPA cisterns (5) close to the 7/8 bundle (4), running into the meatus (→) of the petrosal bone (3). The signal of the pons (6) is overlaid by a spatula artifact (*). The tentorium (2) marks the cranial border of the scan

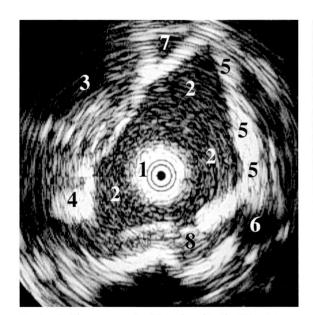

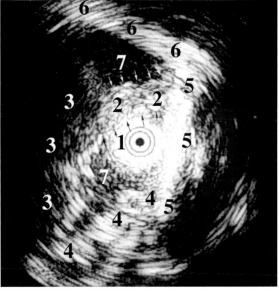

Fig. 3.115. The sono-probe (1) is placed in the CPA cisterns (2), where the tentorium (5) meets the transverse sinus (6), bending into the sigmoid sinus (8). Medially the brain stem is visible with Bochdalek's body (plexus) (4) and the pons (3) where the trigeminal nerve emerges (7)

Fig. 3.116. The sono-probe (1) is placed in the cerebello-pontine cistern (7) between the trigeminal nerve (2 ↑↑↓↓) and the 7/8 bundle (4) and close to the petrosus bone (5) and the surface of the pons (3). The tentorium (6) forms the superior border of the scan

3

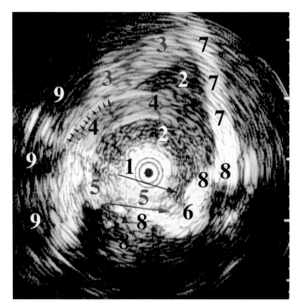

Fig. 3.117. The sono-probe (*1*) is now in the cerebellopontine cistern (*2*) close to the 7/8 bundle (*5*), which runs (→) to the meatus (*6*) in the petrosus bone (*8*). The ICA loop (*4*) is visible, and the compression side (←) at the trigeminal nerve (*3*), where it enters the pons (*9*). The tentorium (*7*) is cut by the scan, but both the transverse and the sigmoid sinus are clearly visible only on the video clip, where the blood flow shows where they are

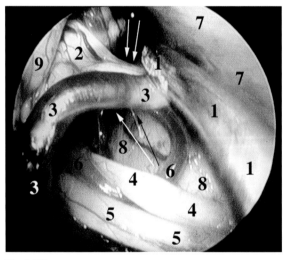

Fig. 3.113.

Vascular Lesions (Fig. 3.118)

Owing to the imaging of blood flow, vessels are well visible in the sono-scan. They can even be seen through the walls of the ventricular system while invisible to the endoscope (Figs. 3.119–3.121).

Aneurysms are detected within a blood clot by visualizing the flow inside the sac, presenting turbulence, and also from the size of the neck. In this way the patency of the parent vessels can be confirmed by a real-time imaging method (Figs. 3.120, 3.121).

Cavernomas are precisely reflected and localized because of their strong echo signal. Even small remnants will be recognized, as will external shape and internal structure and architecture.

In this preliminary series there were no cases with angiomas.

Vascular lesions can be examined in different ways, because their blood flow is well detected by the real-time image of the sono-probe (Table 3.5). In two aneurysms the aneurysm flow was exactly visible but was not well documented owing to technical problems with the video chain. Thickness and calcification of the wall and pulsations were demonstrated, and even a peripheral PICA aneurysm was well detected. Vessel examination by imaging showed physiological parameters. Visualization of a medial aneurysm in a blood clot was possible, making safe preparation easier.

A cavernoma in the hypothalamus was precisely delineated and a remnant diagnosed before the procedure was ended. The border separating it from the optic tract and third ventricle was well demonstrated.

Table 3.5. Vascular lesions

Type of vascular lesion	Observations	*n*
Medial aneurysm	Clip, flow in parent vessels	1
Medial aneurysm	SAH, flow in aneurysm, targeting	1
PICA aneurysm distal	SAH, clip, imaging	1
ACA aneurysm left	Flow of rest of aneurysm, clip	1
ICA aneurysm		2
Cavernoma	Hypothalamus	1

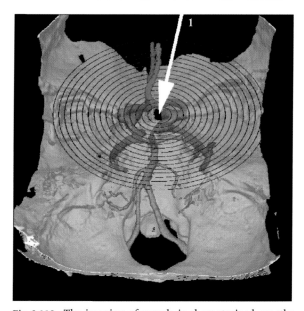

Fig. 3.118. The imaging of vessels is characterized exactly by the blood flow, but confusing at first because of a wide variety of scan shapes, depending upon the course of each vessel through the scan plane. The ENS catheter (1) with the sono-waves now scans the vessel tree transversely

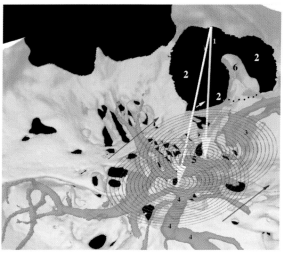

Fig. 3.119. The ENS catheter (1) is now introduced in a right supraorbital approach (2), which is unfinished, as the sphenoid wing (6) is not resected (........). Scanning with the ENS catheter (1) reveals an aneurysm (3) of the M1 bifurcation (*green, yellow*, and *blue*). Its position in the midline close to the basilar artery (4) would not allow the aneurysm to be reached and detected. The change in position (→) to close to the ICA (5) makes scanning of the aneurysm positive. However, such a complex anatomy cannot easily be understood by scanning, and the most important information will be related to flow activity

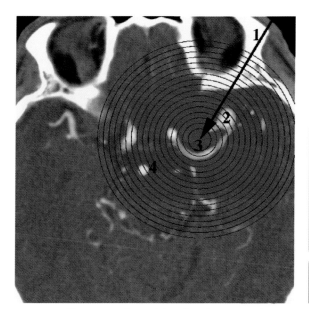

Fig. 3.120. The ENS catheter (1) will only present the vessels (3, 4) that appear in the plane of sono waves. The aneurysm (2) will be cut in slices in such a way that the aneurysm and the bifurcation are not completely represented in one slice, as here

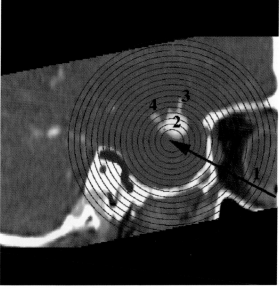

Fig. 3.121. If the direction of the ENS catheter (1) changes from a frontal to a temporal position, the plane of sono-waves will change from axial to sagittal orientation. The shape of the vessels (3, 4) and the slices of the aneurysm (2) will change markedly, and recognition may thus become difficult

3

Case 19

Clinical History

This 43-year-old man had a SAH with ICH on the right side. The hematoma was evacuated and a medial aneurysm clipped. At DAS, a second medial aneurysm on the left side became visible and he was admitted for elective clipping.

The neuroradiological imaging showed a small medial aneurysm of a far dorsal bifurcation on the insula, with a long and wide M1 trunk. In addition, he was found to have an arachnoid cyst in a temporopolar site.

Intraoperatively, the aneurysm was typically directed in the direction of blood flow of the large M1 (Fig. 3.122). The aneurysm was clipped, after which endoscopy revealed a bulging posterior part, so that the clip needed to be corrected.

For technical reasons, the unclipped aneurysm was not caught precisely in the sono-plane, as the approach did not allow the necessary angling of the ENS catheter. However, parent vessels, and the thrombosed aneurysm after clipping, became easily visible in the scan (Figs. 3.123–3.125).

Outcome

The patient subsequently had an uneventful course and recovery after some days of drainage for a subgaleal CSF collection.

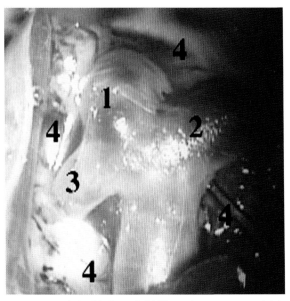

Fig. 3.122. A left-sided medial bifurcation aneurysm (1) is visible with a thick inferior M2 branch (2) plus a smaller superior M2 branch (3), within the sylvian cistern (4)

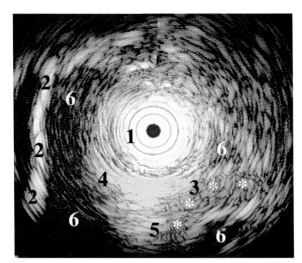

Fig. 3.123. The sono-probe (1) is now placed in the sylvian cistern (6) close to the media bifurcation with the thick inferior M2 branch (3), represented by the blood flow (***). Tangentially scanned, a small superior M2 branch (4) and the M1 trunk (5) can be seen. The aneurysm is not in the scanning plane, except for a small cortical vessel (2) of the frontal operculum

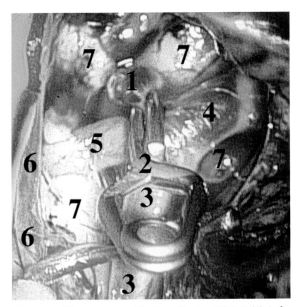

Fig. 3.124. The aneurysm (1) after clipping (2). M1 (3), inferior M2 (4), and superior M2 (5) are visible in the wide open sylvian fissure (7). A small fronto-opercular vessel (6) is also seen

Case 20

Clinical History

This 69-year-old woman had experienced an acute decline of hearing some years before. Finally, the hearing deficit stayed at a constant low level, and neuroradiological investigations were done. MR led to the suspicion of a vascular pathology, and angiography showed an aneurysm of the A1 segment (Fig. 3.126).

Treatment and Outcome

Interventional therapy was not successful, and an operation was indicated. ENS imaging was able to follow the branches of the ICA (Fig. 3.127).

After placement of two clips, ENS still detected a flow signal in the dome of the aneurysm, which the examiner found incredible (Fig. 3.128). However, a gush of blood (Fig. 3.129) followed puncture of the aneurysm, and the clipping had to be corrected.

The patient left 9 days after the operation with a normal neurological status.

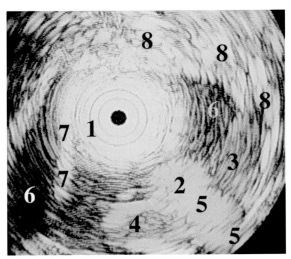

Fig. 3.125. The sono-probe (1) is in contact with the clipped aneurysm (2) without a flow effect inside. The superior (3) and inferior (4) M2 branches are just in the scan, and the M1 trunk is covered by the clip artifact (5). The sylvian cistern (6) and an arachnoid membrane (7) are present. The temporal lobe parenchyma (8) is also scanned

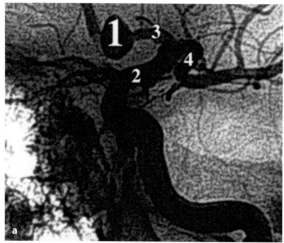

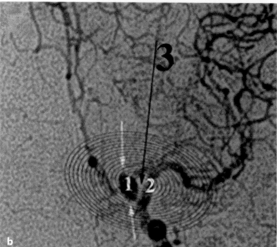

Fig. 3.126. a DSA shows an A1 aneurysm (*1*), which is in quite an atypical location along the course of the carotid artery (*2*), anterior cerebral artery (*3*), and medial cerebral artery (*4*). b The view from above represents the position of the ENS catheter (*3*) with sono-waves (()) cutting the aneurysm (*1*) and the ICA bifurcation (*2*). Both a the oblique view and b the a-p view show the bulge (↓↑) of the aneurysm

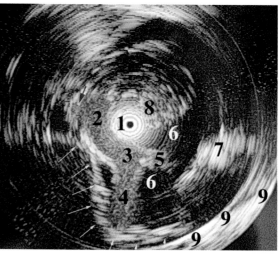

Fig. 3.127. The sono-probe (*1*) is between the left ICA (*2*) and the optic nerves (*8*). The bifurcation (*3*) into A1 (*5*) and M1 (*4*) within the subarachnoid space (*6*), and even branching of Pcom (↓), can be seen. The aneurysm is not within the scan plane, but the clip artifact (*7*), the artifact of a subfrontal spatula (*9*), and the arachnoid membrane of the basal cistern (→) are recognizable

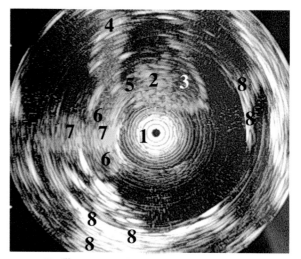

Fig. 3.128. The sono-probe (*1*) is now positioned superior to the bifurcation of ICA (*4*) close to M1 (*6*) and A1 (*5*), nearly in contact with the aneurysm (*2*), in which a flow (*3*) is visible though clips (*7*) have been placed. Artifacts of both subfrontal and temporal spatulas (*8*) are present

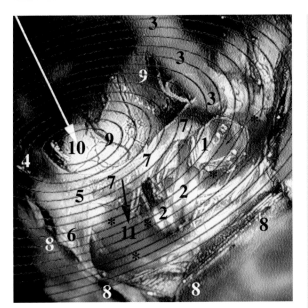

Fig. 3.129. Though two clips (*2*) were placed on the aneurysm's neck (*1*), after puncture (↓) it started to bleed (*) and the clips had to be corrected by suction control (*3*). The sono-scan (()) detected the flow in the clipped aneurysm (see Fig. 3.128). The view under the microscope presents left ICA (*4*), bifurcation (*5*), M1 (*6*), and A1 (*7*) with the aneurysm (*1*). The optic chiasm (*10*) is visible and subfrontal, as is the temporal spatula (*8*). The ENS catheter was positioned inferior (*10*) and superior (*11*) to A1 (*7*)

Case 21

Clinical History

This 53-year-old man had a large SAH IV with ICH in the right frontal lobe. The ICA aneurysm was coiled, and a shunt became necessary. A second non-bleeding ICA bifurcation aneurysm on the left side was untouched, and after the patient recovered from his severe bleeds and from the operation the left aneurysm was clipped (Fig. 3.130).

ENS imaging was able to show the aneurysm and the flow into it (Fig. 3.131). The continuation of the aneurysm and the parent vessels were not in the same plane, and it became difficult to reproduce images showing everything together in one slice (Fig. 3.132).

Outcome

The patient had no additional neurological deficit and went on to rehabilitation therapy.

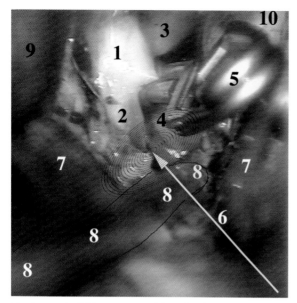

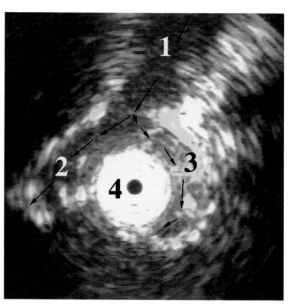

Fig. 3.130. An ICA aneurysm (*4*) at the division of the left ICA (*1*) into the medial cerebral artery (*2*) and anterior cerebral artery (*3*), marked by the aneurysm clip (*5*), is examined by means of the ENS catheter (*6*) with sono-waves and is visible here. A spatula (*7*) is placed on both the temporal lobe (*9*) and the frontal lobe (*10*)

Fig. 3.131. The sono-probe (*4*) is placed close to the bifurcation of ICA (*1*) in the medial cerebral artery (*2*) and flow (↓) into the aneurysm (*3*). The anterior cerebral artery is invisible in the sono-plane

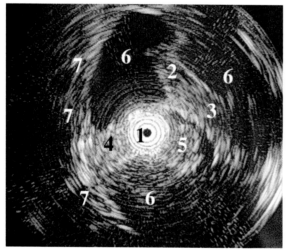

Fig. 3.132. The sono-probe (*1*) is in the subarachnoid space at ICA (*2*), branching in the anterior cerebral artery (*3*) and, though not completely visible in the scan, the medial cerebral artery (*4*). Only the dome of the aneurysm (*5*) is visible. The temporal lobe (*7*) is left sided

Case 22

This illustrative case shows targeting of remnants in the deep tissue, with high resolution in a cavernoma.

Clinical History

This 60-year old women was admitted with headaches and sight problems while reading. An existing arterial hypertonia was already known. The MR scan showed a lesion in the hypothalamus with irregular vessels nearby. Angiography did not confirm the presence of an AVM. The final neuroradiological diagnosis was cavernoma.

Treatment and Outcome

The operation was done from a right pterional approach, and the cavernoma was found medial to the optic tract anterior and posterior to A1. Endoscopic inspection of the resection cavity with additional endosonography showed a remnant of the cavernoma (Figs. 3.133–3.135), which was then resected. The resection was controlled intraoperatively by ENS (Fig. 3.135), and the sella with the pituitary gland was imaged at the same time (Fig. 3.136). A postoperative MR showed complete resection of the lesion.

The postoperative course was excellent, and the patient went home on the 9th day after her operation.

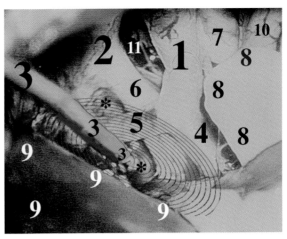

Fig. 3.133. Here the ENS catheter (3) is introduced under microscopic control into the resection cavity (*) of a cavernoma in the hypothalamus from a right pterional approach. The sono-waves (()) are demonstrated. Frontal spatula (9) and temporal brain parts (8) allow viewing of carotid artery (1) and optic nerve (2), A1 (3), M1 (4), Lilliequist membrane (11), and anterior clinoid process (7)

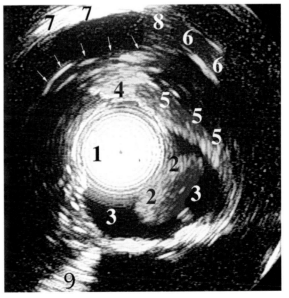

Fig. 3.134. The sono-probe (1) is introduced into the resection cavity (3) of the cavernoma, targeting a remnant (2). The cavity is bordering on the optic tract (5), and the optic nerve (4), ICA (8), M1 (6), and A1 (↓) are also visible. There is an instrument artifact caused by an aspirator (9)

3

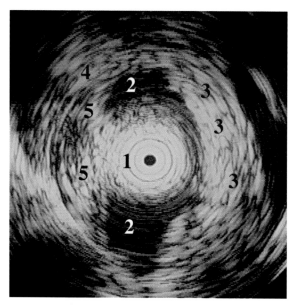

Fig. 3.135. After complete resection of the cavernoma the sono-probe (*1*) is again introduced into the resection cavity (*2*), revealing no remnant at all. The optic tract (*3*) gives a strong signal at the lateral wall of the cavity (*2*). The medial wall is formed by the hypothalamus (*5*), the anterior border being marked by optic chiasm (*4*)

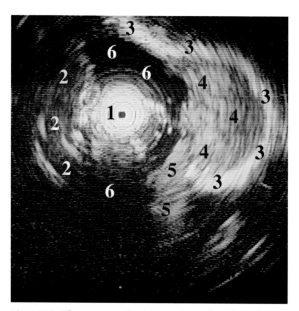

Fig. 3.136. The sono-probe (*1*) was introduced semisagittally from the right pterional into the prechiasmatic window, reaching the suprasellar space (*6*), where the contralateral infraclinoidal and suboptic left ICA (*2*) is detected. The sella (*3*) is also seen, with the pituitary gland (*4*) and pituitary stalk (*5*). The resection cavity was not visible with this approach

Lesions Examined

Miscellaneous lesions are examined, and the largest group was that of intracerebral hematomas.

Ventricular hematomas could be well approached, even in the dark field of endoscopic vision. Safe and almost complete evacuation was possible, with the border between hematoma and ventricular wall being visualized by the sono-scan and giving exact online orientation in all cases. All ventricular hematomas were soft, and the near-complete evacuation meant that one drainage catheter was sufficient and involved no danger of obliteration.

Intracerebral hemorrhages were partially evacuated, and it was possible to check the evacuation and orientation in the dark hematoma precisely with the aid of ENS. Actual bleeds became clearly visible through detection of blood jets and turbulence. In cases of hard hematoma mass, normalization of raised ICP at least was obtained in all cases. The transendoscopic ultrasound aspirator was not available at that time.

Resection Control, Targeting and Navigation

In 39 cases *intraoperative imaging* was the main reason for the investigation, while in 13 *neuronavigation* was the focus of interest. When *tumor resection was to be checked*, even if there were no particular navigation problems the problem of targeting a remnant that had already been visualized still had to be overcome. In 18 imaging cases, targeting a previously imaged lesion or an area of interest was necessary and was successfully achieved.

Table 3.6. Investigations performed and number of cases in which each was used

Investigation	*n*
Imaging	39
Targeting	18
Navigation	13

ewfw[object Object]

Case 23: A Difficult Case Without ENS

Clinical History

After postpartal bleeds this 3-year-old boy was found to have multicystic hydrocephalus with recurrent cystic formations. Multiple shunts had been placed with several catheters in the past, leaving the marks typically seen on our youngest patients (Figs. 3.137, 3.138). Because of the high protein titer of the CSF the shunt systems were frequently obstructed. This little boy had had 27 operations and multiple spinal punctures for examination of the CSF. There had also been several shunt infections. Symptoms varied from high ICP with a typical course to neuropsychological symptoms with changed behavior and activity.

Treatment and Outcome

The operation had to be done as an emergency, and ENS equipment was not available. However, it was possible to place seven perforations between several cysts and into basal cisterns: from the left-sided coronal burr hole, four perforations were performed and one shunt system was explanted under endoscopic control. A parietal burr hole was also made, through which three perforations were placed and a second shunt system was removed endoscopically. Because of the difficult anatomical situation orientation was not easy, and the whole procedure took some 3 hours. It was estimated that with the aid of ENS the whole procedure would have taken no more than 1 hour. In addition, one cyst was not found and caused enlargement 3 weeks after this operation, making it necessary to reshunt the ventricles to prevent raised ICP. However, the shunting did not lead to correction of the neuropsychological symptoms caused by the midline cyst, which was not found without ENS navigation.

After these multiple perforations, the boy did rather well postoperatively, and MR showed the perforations with new flow pathways (Fig. 3.139–3.141). No collapse of the brain or pneumatocephalus was encountered. However, as mentioned above, after 3 weeks the boy developed raised ICP and the midline cyst was enlarged. The communication of all other cysts and ventricles was maintained, and puncture to obtain CSF for investigation was no longer necessary. The multicystic system was simplified by the new CSF communications.

If another shunt complication should appear in the future, we plan to perform an ENS-guided endoscopic procedure to allow communications between the midline cyst and the basal cisterns.

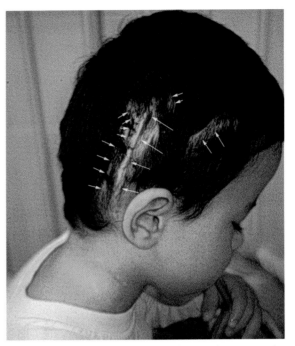

Fig. 3.137. This is a typical aspect of multiple scars on the right posterior side of the head of this 3-year-old boy. Both frontal areas and left posterior area of his head looked similar

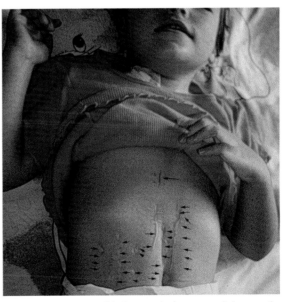

Fig. 3.138. Case 24. This is a typical aspect of thoracoabdominal scars, following multiple shunt revisions. After one endoscopic third ventriculocisternostomy the girl is now shunt free. As in case 23, ENS was not available

3

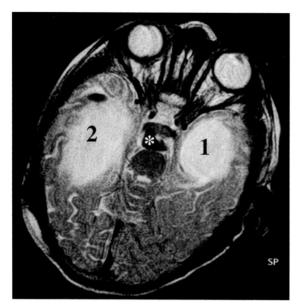

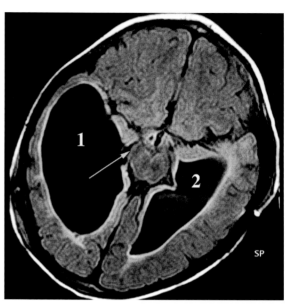

Fig. 3.139. After multiple intercystic and cystocisternal perforations, there is a strong flow signal (*) in the interpeduncular cistern, demonstrated in the postoperative MR, at the pontine level. The left (*1*) and right (*2*) temporal horns were isolated preoperatively and are now smaller following the construction of a communication allowing CSF flow

Fig. 3.140. Postoperative MR at the level of the mesencephalon demonstrates the temporal ventriculo(*1*)-interpeduncular cisternostomy window (→). The isolated left temporal horn (*2*) was released in size by posteromedial perforation

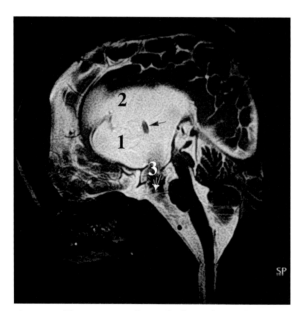

Fig. 3.141. The postoperative sagittal MR shows a huge cyst (*1*) between the lateral (*2*) and third (*3*) ventricles. There is a flow signal from a cystoventriculostomy (←). The strong flow signal (*thick arrow*) in the interpeduncular cistern is not from an ETV but from the right-sided temporo-ventriculo-interpeduncular cisternostomy. The moving floor of the third ventricle is mimicking the flow of an ETV

Summary and Final Reflections

To sum up the clinical results of transendoscopic ultrasound imaging in neurosurgery, we can conclude that while in other fields a great deal of experience has already been collected (see Chap. 1), in neurosurgery we are still just on the threshold. We have one additional benefit of intraoperative imaging over all other disciplines using transendoscopic ultrasound, which is the neuronavigation capacity.

The routine use of ENS has shown the capabilities of this technique in different lesions and problems and highlighted its benefits and limitations. The cases above provide illustrations of most groups of lesions. Table 3.7 gives a summary overview of the applications of ENS. Practical work has made it clear how surprisingly many different applications there are.

The use of additional sono-scanning in endoscopy and microsurgery has made most of the procedures safer or easier. It has been rewarding to see how, once the learning period is over (best done in the laboratory; see chap. 2), endoscopy becomes safer. Moreover, if the sono-catheter is not available endoscopy is more time consuming and the lack of sonographic information in difficult cases leaves the user in an uncomfortable position.

The *shallow penetration* of ENS is a problem, giving sight of only a limited region. In large regions of interest, CT and MR will give a complete view. The catheter has to be moved through the whole field to monitor resection and evacuation.

Strong background signals may overlay the image with a texture that limits interpretation. However, this is also the case in the pixel and voxel world of CT and MR, and imaging resolution is in any case higher in ENS, especially for moving structures.

Geometric torsion by radial scan is a repetitive phenomenon and is soon understood with training. When the angulation of the scanning planes is used torsion may make interpretation difficult at times. Learning becomes easier when the orthogonally defined planes of CT or MR are kept to, thus making correlation easier. The selection of each plane also offers some imaging advantages.

The *protrusion of the probe tip* into the scan plane must be kept in mind and factored into calculations, which means strict observation of the endoscope, including observation by microscope in freehand use.

Sonography, in general, needs a clear field under fluid or by direct tissue contact. Gas insufflation by CSF release results in an *air artifact* or total lack of any image at all.

Conventional sono-scanners 'sound' forward, while the ENS catheter 'sounds' radially and laterally, as if it were a 'brain radar.' Therefore, it is *not possible* to *target a structure in a straight working direction*. This must be calculated during the planning stage. Further developments will soon overcome this (Table 3.8).

Some artifacts are encountered *in the images*, which must be known. They do not always disturb or change the image, but may at times be helpful in orientation and adjustment:

Table 3.7. Treatments and problems, and help provided by endonuclear sonography (*ENS*)

Treatment	Problem	Advantage of ENS
Third ventriculocisternostomy	Localization of basilar artery/perforation	Visualization through floor of third ventricle
Septostomy	Perforation point	Navigation, targeting
Catheter placement	Small ventricle	Navigation
Catheter deletion	Bleeding	Compensation of poor vision
Ventricular hematoma evacuation	Poor sight	Compensation of poor vision, orientation, monitoring of evacuation
ICB evacuation	No landmarks	Compensation of poor vision
	Dark view	Evacuation control
	Difficult orientation	Navigation in the dark
Resection control	Remnant of tumor	Tumor echo and location
Biopsy	Detection of lesion	Navigation
Cystostomy	Orientation	Navigation
Aneurysm clipping	Blood clot, aneurysmal wall	Flow, targeting

Table 3.8. Limitations and implications

Limitation	Consequence/solution
Little penetration depth (radius)	3 cm parenchyma, 6 cm bone
High background signal	Interpretation only >0.5 mm
Geometrical torsion by radial scan	Experience necessary
Geometrical torsion by extraplanar scan	Experience necessary
Tip protrusion 1 mm ahead to scan plane	Planning and visual control
No image in air	Irrigation, clear working field
No scan in anterior direction	Planning, future research

An *air artifact* is an area of no imaging and can be only a segment or comprise a whole radius. It occurs when there are air bubbles in front of the probe inside the sheath or intracranially, or when the probe comes into air. Air artifacts such as air bubbles, however, reflect the surrounding area and can mimic a tumor mass. This could appear in the endoscope image as an irregular mass with bubbles in the CSF acting in the same way as a mirror.

A *metal artifact* produces a sound shadow originating from the instruments used, such as spatulas or clips. Such artifacts do not only disturb the imaging, but can also be helpful in targeting and orientation.

A *rotation artifact* occurs when the rotation of the catheter in the sheath is decelerated by force. Radial beams disturb the image, and the whole image may even rotate, making new adjustment of the orientation necessary.

A special effect is the *lens artifact*, which represents the tip of the endoscope as a strong echo circle, mimicking an axial scan of a vessel.

Indications

A variety of indications have to be discussed.

Ventricular puncture is usually not a problem, but becomes one if the ventricles are small or there is some shifting, or as a result of a change in normal endoscopic anatomy (Perneczky et al. 1993). In these cases use of a simple imaging technique to solve the problem, rather than stereotaxy or neuronavigation, seems justified (Hopf et al. 1998). The usual ultrasound technique is adequate in areas that are not too deep (Rieger et al. 1996). For deep-seated lesions ENS

is far superior to the more common sectoral sonoprobes in terms of optical resolution of the depth.

Ventriculocisternostomy (ETV) is one of the main indications in ENS that still present some problems, such as patency of the ETV stoma, visual control, and criteria for recognizing when it is indicated (Fukuhara et al. 2000; Kulkarni et al. 2000; Reddy et al. 1989; Tisell et al. 2000). However, there are reports of fatal or near-fatal complications in such cases (Handler et al. 1994; Lowry et al. 1996; McLaughlin et al. 1997; Schroeder et al. 1999). The sono-catheter makes orientation and navigation with the endoscope safer by additional real-time imaging and high optical resolution.

Fenestration of cysts may become a problem when they are small, located intraparenchymatously or inside small ventricles, or multiple. Such cases present a navigation problem, which has not yet been solved by current neuronavigation systems (Caemaert et al. 1992; Hopf et al. 1998; Schroeder and Gaab 1998). With the aid of the sono-catheter these lesions can be treated much more easily and safely with a minimum of effort. Especially in close proximity to vessels or important neurological structures, the additional imaging makes the risk calculable, owing to online observation.

Tumor biopsy is difficult in small or deep-seated lesions. In the case of intraventricular cases the release of CSF can cause shifting, and neuronavigation is then unreliable (Tronnier et al. 1999; Wirtz et al. 1997). A combination with stereotaxy is possible, especially if the imaging is insufficient because of a low-echo signal or limited experience (Froelich et al. 1996). If the tumor gives a strong echo signal, as in the case of metastases, the sono-catheter can target the lesion in real time.

It is well known that *aneurysms* are challenging and high-risk lesions (Yasargil 1984a, b). There are many items of information that the sono-catheter can display about them, which again can make the approach easier. Blood flow before and after clipping, an aneurysm inside a blood clot, a thrombosis inside an aneurysm, the constitution of an aneurysmal wall, and the intraluminal result of vessel reconstruction by clipping can all be seen online. This information cannot be obtained by endoscopy alone (Perneczky and Fries 1998; Taniguchi et al. 1999) and is dependent on regular postoperative control by means of DSA, MRA, or CTA. The intraoperative information provides an opportunity for direct correction if needed.

Neuronavigation has come into quite wide use, but it has yet to be determined whether its benefits justify the investment it entails in terms of effort and cost

Table 3.9. Indications/solutions

Indication	Solution
Ventricular puncture	Navigation + subependymal target
Ventriculocisternostomy	Transventricular imaging of intepeduncular cistern
Fenestration of cysts	Navigation + imaging of size
Tumor resection control	High-resolution imaging intraoperatively
Tumor biopsy	Targeting + bleeding control
ICH evacuation	Evacuation control, navigation
Aneurysm examination	Neck, rupture side, pulsation, etc.
Endoneuronavigation	Sono-navigated neuroendoscopy in real time, simple, not expensive

(Fahlbusch and Nimsky 2000; Kelly 2000; Levy 1998; Maciunas 2000; Shekhar 2000; Wirtz et al. 1997) Moreover, some 'navigation' systems do not fulfill the true definition of navigation, as they lack real-time feedback, which the sono-catheter facilitates by providing real-time and online intraoperative imaging with true navigation capabilities. As indicated above, the sono-catheter can solve most navigation problems in neuroendoscopy with a minimum of effort and at low cost. Moreover, the sono-catheter can assist in microneurosurgery as an intraoperative imaging tool.

There are two indications that have not yet been examined but are possible application candidates according to the laboratory results:

- *Morphometric ICP monitoring* at the bedside by imaging of ventricular sizes and changes.
- *Bedside imaging of space-occupying lesions*, such as *tumors* and *hematomas*, as a *substitute for CT* in ICU patients.

With regard to the enormous logistic and financial effort involved in diagnostic imaging in ICU patients, the last two suggested indications, which have still not been investigated, could have a significant impact on the healthcare system: the technique comes to the patient and not vice versa.

The concept of bedside diagnosis and therapy will be a great benefit to the patient as well as to the healthcare system. Thus, there is a convergence of interests and needs (Table 3.9).

Future developments of ENS will depend on more documentation and analysis of clinical results. This experience should give a user profile for better adaptation of the system to the needs of neurosurgery. Display of physiological parameters and real-time 3D reconstruction, which are now possible with general sonography, should also be developed for ENS. Combination with other techniques, such as laser navigation or the neuronavigation interface, may make new applications and easier interpretation possible.

ENS is not just a tool; it may rather become the cornerstone of a new concept behind a new technical generation of neurosurgery. This concept will be presented in chapter 5. The ultimate goal of ENS is to assist in minimizing the trauma to our patients by ergonomic real-time imaging (Figs. 3.142, 3.143).

A list of investigations for the future is displayed in Table 3.10.

Table 3.10. Topics for further studies

More clinical evaluation and experience
Enhanced adaptation to neurosurgery
3-D ENS in real time
Better integration of physiological parameters
Compatibility with other techniques
List of approved indications
Probes with forward sound direction
Integration into a general design of miniaturization
ENS courses for training in the new technique

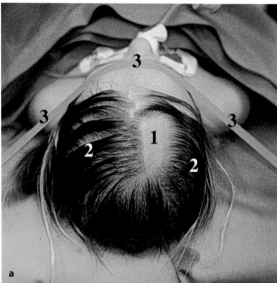

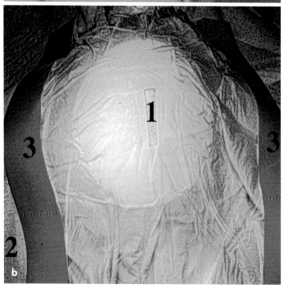

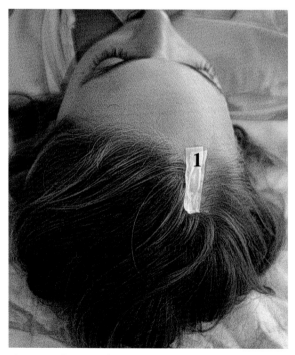

Fig. 3.142. a To keep the overall trauma low, a small area is shaved (*1*). For the same reason, colorless disinfection of the skin together with all the hair (*2*) and simple fixation of the head with drapes (*3*) were performed. b Only a small area of skin was exposed (*1*), with close draping (*2*) and additional fixation with foil (*3*), and this was sufficient

Fig. 3.143. Case 25: view on 1st postoperative day, showing the cosmetic result (*1*) of the minimally invasive technique, which is essential for a short and favorable postoperative course, especially in our youngest patients

Conclusions

In terms of lowering the level of risk in brain surgery further, ENS appears to be a desirable and useful tool in the hands of experienced neurosurgeons, being relatively low cost and easy to apply.

The importance of the stage of laboratory training must not be underestimated; this, however, will pay off handsomely in the form of added confidence and better results in the operating room. It will release surgeons from a multitude of tasks that currently fall to them, and this combination of simplicity and added safety warrants further exploitation of the merits of the technique and the possibilities it offers.

In summary, ENS is a tool for:
- Intraoperative real-time and online high-resolution imaging
- Neuronavigation of endoscopes with a working channel at least 2 mm in diameter
- Making neuroendoscopy easier and safer
- Application in a wide variety of indications
ENS is:
- Small, mobile and easy applicable in endo- and microneurosurgery
- Limited by the need for laboratory work and clinical experience
- Open to further development
- A cornerstone of a new concept of MIN (see chapter 5)

ENS Clips

DVD

4

Contents

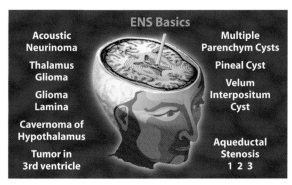

Fig. 4.1. Start-Interface DVD

Laboratory Work: Setting

The rapid evolution of neurosurgical techniques has led to the need for new surgical and mental skills, which need to be practiced in laboratory work. Present-day knowledge of ergonomics, neuropsychology, and complexity analysis explains why virtual methods of training are not enough and only training models that are close to surgery can have any relevant benefit. The whole topic of training needs in neurosurgery has recently been opened up to a new discussion.

This training model was created in 1986 and is applied within 3 days after a death. It has proved to be a valuable training model for endoscopy-assisted microneurosurgery.

Animal training is important as a training tool only insofar as it offers the experience of dealing with living tissue. This, however, is not the main problem for surgeons; their main difficulty, as described above, lies in implementing mental and physical

Clip no.	Case no.	Diagnosis	Indication
		Laboratory	Equipment and anatomy
1	1	Aqueductal stenosis	ETV, Imaging 3-D Imaging
2	29	Multiple parenchymal cysts	Cyst fenestration
3	22	Acoustic neurinoma	Imaging
4	37	Thalamus – glioma	Imaging, tumor borders
5	36	Pineal cyst	Imaging, tumor, cyst (?)
6	47	Aqueductal stenosis, Monro stenosis	Septostomy, ETV, targeting
7	38	Tumor in third ventricle	Imaging, ETV
8	40	Glioma lamina quadrigemina	Imaging
9	44	Velum interpositum cyst	Targeting, navigation
10	42	Aqueductal stenosis	Imaging, ETV
11	13	Cavernoma of hypothalamus	Imaging, targeting

ergonomics in neurosurgery. This cannot be learned in animal-based training, because the 'gestalt' phenomena cannot be fulfilled by training on animals. The neuropsychological process encountered in an animal training model is too far removed from that experienced during surgery on a human cranium. Recognition and the implications for manual procedures in human surgery are too different from those in animal training. Approach analysis and approach design, surgical strategy, and neuropsychological environment in human surgery cannot be simulated in animal models.

In our laboratory setting dissections were done within 4–72 hours after death. Modern neurosurgical techniques were applied at the dissection table, so that the operating microscope, a range of endoscopes and video techniques, and various sonography machines, microsurgical instruments, and items of bipolar and suction equipment were available. The setting is comparable to a surgical one, and our focus of interest was the simulation of live surgery with minimally invasive techniques. In some cases, computer-assisted planning was done in addition. The tissue used was not fixed, and no vessels were injected. The cranium was never disconnected, but the whole body was positioned as if for surgery.

This laboratory model can give training in:

- Understanding anatomical topography
- Analysing of imaging findings
- Analysing approaches (approach planning)
- Cisternal preparation
- Paraendoscopic methods (video surgery)
- Analysing the ergonomics of the setting and the instrumentation
- Manual skills and mental training according to the principles of neuropsychology

Anatomical Cases (with PIP)

Ventriculoscopy

Though vision through the endoscope is impaired by ependymal tissue (PIP), the position of the sono-probe in the right frontal horn of the lateral ventricle can be accurately recognized, representing the position of the tip of the endoscope. In parallel with this, the tip of the sono-catheter can be controlled visually in the endoscopic view. The frontal falx, the pellucid septum, and the contralateral frontal horn are visible in the sono-view.

An air bubble in the fluid of the superior corner of the frontal horn is not recognized endoscopically because it mirrors the surrounding tissue. However, it is still diagnosed, because the sono-image presents an air artifact.

When we start from this position the localization of the foramen of Monro is not visible in the endoscopic view but is already present in the sono-view, making it possible to steer the scope to that target by real-time online imaging. The position of the endoscope at the pellucid septum and in relation to the contralateral frontal horn is visible, so that a perforation point can be defined for septostomy.

Suprasellar Space

The sono-catheter is advanced under endoscopic control (PIP) and placed between the two optic nerves in front of the chiasm and superior to the diaphragm of the sella. The semi-sagittal scan of the sono-image shows many structures that are not visible in the endoscopic view (PIP): the entire parenchyma of the pituitary gland is visible, with pituitary stalk and sella. The optic chiasm, the lamina terminalis, and the anterior third ventricle can be seen.

As the catheter is moved under the left optic nerve it is scanned and becomes visible in the sono-view.

Fourth Ventricle

The endoscopic view in the PIP is directed into the fourth ventricle, showing the choroid plexus and rhomboid cephalon. The sono-image presents a view into the parenchyma around the ventricle, with the typical pentagonal shape familiar from CT and MR.

As the sono-catheter is advanced under endoscopic control to the left foramen of Luschka (PIP) the sono-image presents the choroid plexus passing through the foramen into the CPA.

Clip 1: First Clinical Case (with PIP; ENS-navigated ETV)

The first clinical test shows the endoscopically controlled advancement of the sono catheter into the third ventricle. The sono-scan presents the level of the foramen of Monro. Following further advancement the typical anatomy of the third ventricle is seen and the sono-view also presents the contralateral foramen of Monro with the pulsating plexus in the liquor.

After perforation of the premamillary membrane (floor of the third ventricle), in the endoscopic view recognition is impaired by floating membranes while the anatomy of the interpeduncular cistern is already seen in the sono-image. The basilar artery and its blood flow are visible, and as the sono-catheter is advanced further the superior cerebellar arteries and the dorsum of the sella also come into view. All these anatomical structures allow precise navigation of the scope before the endoscope can make these structures visible in addition.

3-D Reconstructions (Figs. 2.60–2.62)

With the aid of a 3-D workstation the sono-scans can be converted to 3-D images and displayed on a monitor. In the first case a third ventriculocisternostomy done with the sono-catheter is shown in a coronal view. Elective parameters are set to cause the 3-D reconstruction to move at a selected speed and angle. The scan plane is shown on the right and the 3-D version, on the left. The sono-catheter passes through the frontal horn, along the septum, through the foramen of Monro into the third ventricle, and then along the basal cistern into the foramen magna.

The second clip of a clinical case shows a sagittal plane view of the same procedure.

Clinical Cases

Clip 2: Parenchymal Multiple Cyst, Parietal Right Side (Imaging, Targeting, Navigation)

MR shows a triplanar view of two parietal cysts with a paraventricular presentation, which have shifted only minimally relative to their size. The smaller cyst produces higher intensity than the large one. Such intraparenchymal cysts make it difficult to find the optimal target point for perforation. It was decided to fenestrate both cysts into the lateral ventricle and to take histology specimens.

We start at the point where the tip of the sono-probe reaches the wall of the larger cyst, pushing it away from the parenchyma. The endoscope shows nothing but the white appearance of the white matter. A small gap is growing, and at the moment of perforation an air artifact caused by irrigation is visible. Endoscopic vision is not clear, as the cyst wall tissue is still covering the lens of the endoscope.

Once inside the cyst we are confronted with the typical intraparenchymal problem of orientation, as the wall has no transparency. Is the bulging area the small cyst? The sono-probe can be used to scan this finding, whether or not the endoscope is moved.

The sono-scan makes diagnosis of both the large and the small cyst possible, and also allows recognition of the lateral ventricle with the choroid plexus, which gives a strong echo signal. Under endosonographic control a forceps is used to open up the small cyst and specimens are taken for histology.

The perforation of the small cyst can be visualized both by endoscopy and by sono-scan after a perforation target into the lateral ventricle is defined. The ventricle is entered close to the glomus of the choroid plexus. The optical resolution of the choroid plexus is demonstrated and focused by the zoom function, showing the pulsations and the tiny villi of the plexus tissue.

In the endoscopic view the perforators of the posterior choroid artery are visible.

Finally a hyperechogenic area appears at the base of the small cyst wall. The contrast change and frequency selected (10–30 MHz) indicate the presence of hyperechogenic tissue, arousing the suspicion of a tumor. This was taken out transendoscopically under targeting control by sono-scan and subjected to histological examination, yielding the diagnosis of astrocytoma (WHO I). This case is also illustrated in chap. 3 (Figs. 3.55–3.57).

Clip 3: Acoustic Neurinoma, Left Side (Imaging)

After lateral suboccipital craniotomy the tumor is inspected endoscopically from the inferior and the superior (tentorial) windows. The aims are to see the anatomical relationship and perhaps get an early view of the facial nerve. The foramen jugular nerve boundle and the tumor form the inferior window. The pons and the abducens nerve are visible, while the superior window allows a view of a double superior petrosal vein.

ENS reveals the tumor mass with a view inside the tumor (mostly between 11 o'clock and 3 o'clock), which appears to be homogeneous. Interestingly, the tumor has almost the same echo-density as the brain tissue (in contrast to meningiomas). The skull base is recognizable by its very high echo-density, and the CFS is characterized by very low (black) echo-density.

4

After tumor resection we see the wide opening of the internal acoustic meatus and the facial nerve within the arachnoid membranes.

The sono-scan, working in the jugular meatus window, presents the 'empty' internal auditory meatus (at 3 o'clock) and the jugular bulb with blood flow inside (at 5 o'clock). In the overview (low zoom) the facial nerve is scanned 'coming out of the meatus and running to the pons' (appearing retrogradely in the scan). Again, the jugular blood flow is scanned and then the trigeminal nerve, working in the meatal tentorial window.

In summary, the tumor and brain tissue, the cranial nerves, and the canals into the skull base are visible, as are the blood flows inside the jugular bulb.

Clip 4: Thalamus Glioma, Third Ventricle (Imaging, ENS-navigated Septostomy)

In this case the sono-catheter is used as a guidewire for the endoscope as the sono-probe is advanced up to the endoscope tip until it presents the typical ventricular scan. Thus, we start with the typical appearance of the right frontal horn and the pellucid septum. Now the endoscope can safely follow and also reaches the ventricle. The tumor is now clearly visible in the foramen of Monro. A small gap between tumor and fornix provides a useful window for the sono-probe to scan the tumor.

After a biopsy specimen is taken there is a small bleed, which can also be seen in the sono-scan. The sono-probe is used as a blunt 'seeing' dissector.

To prevent unilateral obstruction of the CSF flow in the foramen of Monro a septostomy is made with the sono-probe, care being taken to avoid injuring a contralateral ependymal vein. The perforation is controlled online in the sono-scan view. The sono-scope exits through the parenchymal canal, and the sono-scan can then monitor bleeding in the parenchyma, which is not visible by means of the endoscope alone.

Clip 5: Pineal Cyst, Third Ventricle [Imaging, Tumor (?), Borders of the Lesion (?)]

This lesion was diagnosed as a pineal tumor on MR. We start our journey as the sono-probe enters the brain parenchyma of the right frontal lobe, where we recognize the first landmark, which is the falx cerebri. This gives us the orientation for the coordinates in the sono-scan. The falx has to appear on the left of the probe and as a vertical line. This means

that the sono-image can be adjusted and fine-tuning can be achieved, enabling us to use the sono-image for navigation. The further journey leads us into the large frontal horn, and we also see a very thin septum and the large opposite frontal horn. We enter the third ventricle very slowly and stay a while at the level of the foramen of Monro, which is characterized by the transverse band of the choroid plexus running from one foramen to the other in contact with the roof of the third ventricle. As we progress, we see the narrowing of the third ventricle and a cyst appears in the pineal recess.

The specifically endoscopic imaging gives sight into the large ventricular system, starting deep in the posterior third ventricle and revealing a tumor. The journey back shows us all the typical signs of chronic hydrocephalus.

A close-up sono-scan is concentrated on the cyst itself, yielding two findings: the wall is thin, and the content is liquid with the echo-density of cerebrospinal fluid (CSF).

The partial resection and cyst evacuation are accomplished microsurgically and are seen in the microscopic view.

The next sonographic journey starts with the sono-probe at the level of the pineal gland at the entrance to the aqueduct, where the round outline of the cyst is no longer seen. Contrast is low owing to selection of the wrong frequency, but the calcification and the strong echo signal still allow recognition of the pineal gland. Once the aqueduct is crossed the typical structure of the superior vermis of cerebellum can be recognized (at 7 o'clock), after which we enter the fourth ventricle with its typical pentagonal shape. Owing to a low zoom we can also recognize the border of the petrosal bone. On the way back we can see the typical anatomical structures again.

The final endoscopic control starts with the view onto the anterior floor of the third ventricle, with a thin transparent premamillary membrane giving sight of a strong basilar artery trunk. We then follow on into the posterior third ventricle and see the remnant of the cyst wall, but also a free passage into the aqueduct.

Clip 6: Asymmetrical Ventricles, Multiple Shunt Infections (ENS-navigated Septostomy and ETV)

We start this journey with the ENS catheter leading us into the left frontal horn. There are several rotation artifacts, making it necessary to adjust the imaging orientation. After this we enter the left frontal horn by the endoscopic view and see the change caused to the ependyma by several bleeds and infections.

Now we have to decide on the target point for perforation of the septum to overcome the stenosis of the left foramen of Monro. As the left frontal horn is small, the stomy will have to be opposite the small frontal horn on the right side, which cannot be safely made by endoscopy alone. The ENS view tells us easily where it is safe to perforate. The perforation can be followed by sono-imaging online, but again there are rotation artifacts. The ENS catheter is used as a 'seeing dissector' to make the perforation while avoiding damage to the structure on the right side. We can understand intuitively how the ENS view makes the perforation process safer, and we can reproduce the online observation while passing through the septum.

Now we cut sharply to the next sequence, finding the ENS catheter already sited in the interpeduncular cistern by ETV and imaging the basilar tip vessels. With the zoom function we can get a close-up view showing the dark peduncles at 5 and 7 o'clock, and between these the round scan of the basilar artery trunk with the blood flow inside. Scanning the basilar head we see the flow in the P1 segments and the oculomotor nerve. Coming back into the third ventricle we see the P2 segment and the P-com segment.

In the endoscopic view into the prepontine area we see a lot of arachnoid scarring and opaque arachnoid membranes, which are remnants of multiple infections. It is easy to recognize how difficult perforation of such tough membranes can be.

The next sono-view again presents the trunk of the basilar artery and the wall of the prepontine cistern and the clivus. Then we follow the basilar artery up to the vertebrobasilar junction by means of the ENS catheter and see the division of the basilar trunk into the two vertebral arteries. At this level, the clivus becomes typically narrow and concave.

The return to the third ventricle is followed by endoscopy until we pass the vertebrobasilar conjunction, where our journey ends.

Clip 7: ETV (ENS Imaging of Vertebro-basllar System, Tumor Imaging)

This endoscopic journey starts in the right frontal horn and leads us to an enlarged foramen of Monro, through which the floor of the third ventricle

and tumor masses are visible. Inside the third ventricle we see changes to the ependyma. The tumor has infiltrated the intermediate mass and the thalamus. Inspection of the posterior third ventricle shows an exophytically growing part of the tumor, and behind the tumor a clear view into the enlarged suprapineal recess. There, the vena magna cerebri and the left basal vein are visible through the translucent arachnoid membrane of the lamina quadrigeminal cistern. The white mass of the splenium of the corpus callosum is also visible in close proximity to the large veins.

The next sequence illustrates ETV in a case in which there is little space to perform the perforation because of a tough membrane immediately dorsal to the sella. The interpeduncular cistern is finally opened, and there is a view along the basilar artery trunk into the prepontine cistern with typical subarachnoid trabecules.

The ENS tour starts inside the interpeduncular cistern with the clivus as a baseline for orientation, while the basilar artery, in this case at 8–9 o'clock, is hardly recognizable. Then we travel retrogradely back to the third ventricle, recognizing the tumor in the right thalamus and an intermediate mass. There is an artifact caused by an instrument at 2 o'clock close to the sono-probe. Under endoscopic control the sono-catheter scans the tumor, showing its parenchyma and borders. Around the third ventricle the ENS catheter can show parts of the circle of Willis, which are not of course visible by means of the endoscope. Both A1 and CoA are visible at 12 o'clock.

The final way out again passes all the structures in the endoscopic view, and close-up scanning by means of the ENS catheter repeats the view into the tumor parenchyma with fine-tuning, so that even the tumor borders in the thalamus are precisely delineated.

Clip 8: Glioma of Lamina Quadrigemina, Aqueductal Stenosis (ETV, Tumor Imaging)

In this case the journey starts with a mistake, as the adjustment of the endoscopic view is upside-down relative to the real anatomy of the patient. The choroid plexus runs upward, in contrast to the real anatomy; In the next scene the image is correctly adjusted. Now it can be used to navigate the endoscope, and the same is true for the sono-view (see chap. 1). We enter the third ventricle through an enlarged foramen of Monro and immediately recognize the cause of the aqueductal stenosis, which is a tumor obliterating the entrance to the aqueduct.

The following scene shows an ETV in a case in which the basilar head is very close to the dorsum of the sella, and a thin translucent membrane is again very tough. Coagulation was preferred and undertaken at the point where the dorsum of the sella is below, as recommended in such cases. Moreover, this is an example of a basilar tip located rather high, not allowing the membrane to hang low even in the presence of hydrocephalus. This means a major criterion for occlusive hydrocephalus is not met, because it cannot occur in such an anatomical constellation. Note the air bubbles on coagulation and bear in mind how difficult perforation may be; in this case the only way to accomplish it was to use a very soft, blunt 2-F Fogarty catheter. The direction of the perforation is not the same as that of the basilar trunk, but slightly lateral to it. Note how slowly the dilatation is done and how long the dilated balloon is kept in place to avoid bleeding and to allow sufficiently careful observation of the rupturing membrane.

The ENS sequence shows the slight difference in echo-intensity between the tumor and the brain tissue. However, as the ENS catheter can be moved directly to the target it can produce a high-resolution sonography depicting even slight differences in echo-density. It can be seen that a solid tumor is present, and not just a cyst. The sono-catheter is better than MR for differentiation between a cyst and a solid tumor. The ENS catheter can be advanced a long way ahead of the endoscope, so that imaging in the third ventricle is possible when the endoscope is placed in the frontal horn.

A close-up sono-view going back from the third ventricle to the frontal horn ends this journey.

Clip 9 (see chap. 3, case 8, Figs. 3.58–3.64): Arachnoid Cyst in the Velum Interpositum (Cyst Fenestration from Left Occipital Horn)

In this case we start with the positioning of the child, also showing the minimally invasive technique, which begins with minimal shaving of the head hair. No sharp fixation is necessary, especially in children.

From the occipital horn of the left lateral ventricle we start the imaging and see the glomus of the choroid plexus of the trigone area. The cyst wall is extremely elastic. For high precision in navigation

the ENS catheter is kept very close to the tip of the endoscope, causing a working canal artifact if the sono-probe slips inside the canal.

Then we enter the cyst and experience how difficult orientation can be in such cysts, as there are no safe landmarks that can be used. It takes some time to find the perfect site for perforation into the cyst. Even the bulging of the cyst into the ventricle does not provide a safe landmark, as the structures behind it cannot be seen. In this case the wall was coagulated after selection of the perforation target. Entering the cyst again shows up another problem, in the form of poor endoscopic vision inside a cyst owing to inadequate illumination in large cysts or to bleeding or opaque fluid inside the cyst.

There was a hemorrhage into the cyst in this case: coagula could be observed online in the sono-view, while the vision in the endoscope became poor. After bleeding, orientation is impossible inside a cyst or ventricle without a second imaging. For navigation in such circumstances the imaging technique must have real-time and online capabilities, which can be supplied by ENS. Computer-assisted neuronavigation only functions in ventricles and cysts if there is no loss of CSF and no irrigation.

Clip 10; Aqueductal Stenosis (ENS ETV, Sono-imaging Only, Imaging of Circle of Willis)

In this case the endoscopic recording is not present owing to a technical error. However, with the training gained from the cases above it is possible to understand the anatomy from sono-imaging alone. This ventricular sono-journey and ETV can be used to test the experience recorded so far.

We start our journey in the parenchyma, which is reached through a right frontal burr hole. There is no landmark within the parenchyma, but in this case of a hydrocephalic ventricular system, navigation to the frontal horn is no problem. It would be usual to zoom down to see the straight echo-strong line of the falx medially. In this case we suddenly land inside the large right frontal horn, which gives us the landmarks needed to fine-tune the imaging adjustment. The septum first serves for orientation, and in the case of the right frontal horn it must appear medial to the sono-probe. However, the final test of correct imaging is the movement of the endoscope, which must present congruency between reality and the images on the monitor.

Slowly we enter the foramen of Monro, and when we look carefully we can see the blood flow in the thalamostriate vein. Then we see the choroid plexus running to the contralateral foramen and along the roof of the third ventricle. The pellucid septum, the columna of the fornices, and the wide-open contralateral foramen with floating plexus can be seen. Little by little we enter the third ventricle; the shape changes as the sono-probe advances.

The elongated shape of the third ventricle tells us that we are in the middle of the ventricle, when suddenly we recognize vessels around and outside the ventricle. We see the scanning of different parts of the circle of Willis (CW) and the blood flow in these vessels. Of course these vessels cannot be seen in the endoscope. First the anterior part of CW is scanned through the lamina terminalis, both A1 and AcoA being clearly recognizable. After that we come to the posterior part of the third ventricle and CW. The basilar artery, with both P1 segments, the left P2 segment and the left P-com entering the left ICA, is visible from its blood flow. At 12 o'clock we have a major sonographic landmark of the suprasellar region, the echo-intense dorsum of the sella.

The next scene illustrates perforation of the ventricular floor by the sono-probe. The force used to perforate the tough premamillary membrane causes the rotation artifact, with a sudden change of the coordinates. After that we see the classic landmarks of the interpeduncular cistern: the dorsum of the sella and the basilar artery, and the cerebral peduncles. The basilar artery is scanned at the trunk level and the arachnoid membranes are floating.

Clip 11: Hypothalamic Cavernoma (Imaging, Targeting and Resection Control)

Through a right pterional approach we see a tumoral change of the tissue in the right optic tract. There is xanthochromia, and an unusual vein is seen crossing over the right optic nerve. The ENS catheter is used freehand at first, as a 'seeing' dissector, in this case. It can be seen that sonography needs a liquid medium for use. The catheter is inserted lateral to the carotid artery.

The sono-view shows the flow in the vessel and also the wall of the vessel.

Now, under microscopic control, the catheter enters the optic-carotid window through the clear liquid.

The sono-view shows the carotid anatomy and blood flow to the right of the probe and the right

optic nerve tissue to the left. The carotid bifurcation can hardly be seen. After opening up the tumoral tissue we find the cavernoma medial to the optic tract within the right hypothalamus.

Now we change to transendoscopic sonography, which has the additional advantage of continuous rinsing and excellent visualization of both the tissue and the sono-probe. Passing the right A1 segment we find the resection cavity and clear it by endoscopic rinsing. Then we pass laterally from the carotid artery towards the interpeduncular cistern, watching the oculomotor nerve emerging from the deep tissue. Advancing the sono-probe at a level inferior to the hypothalamus allows us to scan the cavernoma site from below. A long way back we again recognize the bifurcation of the carotid artery.

In the sono-view we see the carotid artery from its intraclinoidal part to the bifurcation and the M1 segment disappearing into the sylvian cistern medial to the uncus.

Now we follow the prechiasmatic route towards the sella, scanning the hypothalamus from the anterior side. In the sono-view we recognize the sella and the pituitary gland. The stalk becomes visible, as do the carotid artery on the contralateral side and the anterior third ventricle. Finally we come back along the A1 segment and enter the resection cavity to look for remnants of the cavernoma. We see the small cavity and the sono-probe inside, the optic tract laterally, and the hypothalamus parenchyma medially. At 6 o'clock a discrete echo-dense remnant is recognized.

The preparation is continued toward the remnant direction within the angle of the carotid bifurcation. The final resection control by sono-probe shows the larger resection cavity after evacuation of the residual cavernoma, and sono-imaging does not reveal a remnant. Meticulous control shows the probe within the cavity, the optic tract and the carotid bifurcation with blood flow, and the medial wall of the hypothalamus with the cavity of the third ventricle.

The imaging control route continues into the interpeduncular cistern; however, this part of the trunk of the basilar artery is more easily visible than parts of the resection cavity. Even the basilar head can be seen, but owing to angling limits the hypothalamic region does not come into view.

The final microscopic view shows that minimally invasive imaging with a miniprobe allows easy access through microsurgical and endoscopic approaches.

Chapter 5

Future Concepts for Minimally Invasive Techniques in Neurosurgery

5

Contents

Theoretical environment of ENS

Intelligent Interface: Human–Technical System

There have been decisively inappropriate developments in previous systems, in that attempts have been made to use these systems to solve problems that the human being can actually solve better (or that Nature has solved in some better way). This is because in many cases the combined abilities of humans and machinery are not interpreted as a common system, as long as there is no problem directly caused by the human; if that were the case, there would be an interactive complementary strategy between the abilities of the machine and the abilities of the human being. Only when it is not possible or useful for the human being to be on site are other valid considerations applied, which are then and only then used very extensively and at vast expense (Figs. 5.1, 5.2).

Fig. 5.1. Disintegrated interface design

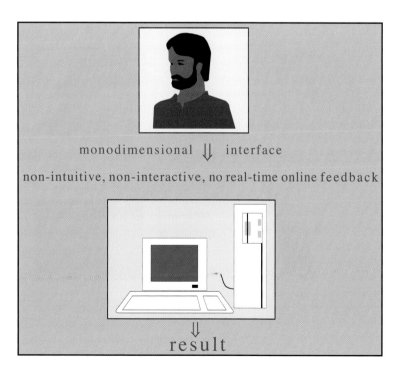

5

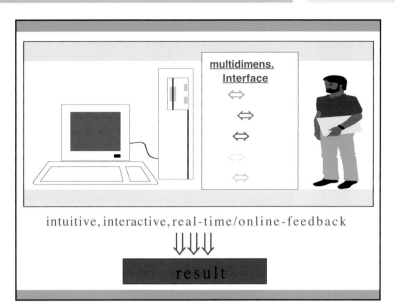

Fig. 5.2. Integrated interface design

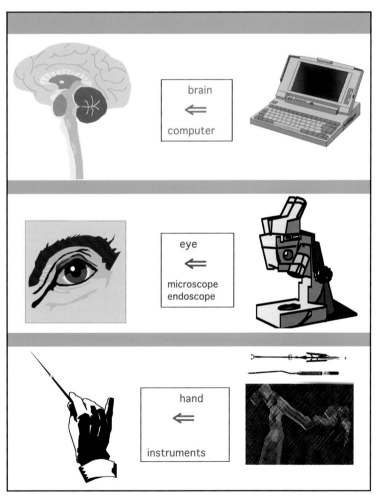

Fig. 5.3. Interfaces: the classic technical supports for human abilities are specifically: for the eyes (microscope or endoscope), the hand (instruments and robotics), and the brain (computers)

For the time being, for example, it does not make sense to attempt to replace the capabilities of the human hand in neurosurgery. This has of course been worthwhile in the prosthesis industry, because in that case the final result is always acceptable, something that is missing being replaced. For the operator, however, every technical system is essentially dependent on the operation of the surgeon's hands, which means that the human hand is unequalled in this case. This statement is often polemically contradicted, with partial individual capabilities, such as accuracy, being selected. However, it is the actual sum and complexity of the abilities of the human hand that make the surgeon's hands so irreplaceable (see Fig. 5.12).

Finding how to solve difficult and relevant problems, instead of trying to find how to replace technically inaccessible human abilities by robotics, for example, has many advantages: to this end, effort is concentrated on optimal solutions to genuine problems, which increases the user's acceptance of the system considerably. It is incomprehensible why anyone might think the abilities of experienced surgeons' hands should be unnecessarily disposed of, particularly when the solution is often worse than the natural variant. Developments in these projects through work devoted to problems of this sort are very expensive and time consuming. The intelligent interface always leads to the result of intuitive and interactive operability. This then increases the rapid learnability and safety of the system and with that, in end-effect, its acceptance (Fig. 5.3).

The main interfaces are:
- Brain (computer, simulation, navigation, monitoring, virtual reality)
- Eye (microscope, endoscope, sonography, intraoperative imaging)
- Hand (instruments, robotics)

Further known interfaces:
- Jaw (mouth-operated switch)
- Foot (foot-operated switch)
- Voice (speech-activated control)

A number of others are possible:
- Pupils
- Electromagnetic field of the brain
- Muscle tension
- Tongue
- Virtual reality (VR) techniques with emerging qualities

Intelligent interface configuration means that the interface must be configured according to the following principles:
- Compatible with neuropsychological principles
- Compatible with technical and mental ergonomics
- Intuitive operability
- Interactive usability (emerging qualities)

Compatible with neuropsychological principles. All that humans do consciously is initiated, controlled, and navigated by their brains. Every activity goes through a neurological process, and conversely, every one of these activities causes a response in the brain. This cybernetic system, with its ancient real-time online feedback mechanism, can only be broken by immense 'power.' Therefore, fundamentally we must strive to adapt technical developments to the principle functions of the brain. Most technical systems do not take any account of this, which means they cannot attain more than moderate acceptance and success.

For the operating surgeon, particular importance attaches to the sensorimotor and the optical subsystems. The special features of these systems must demand proper technical developments, as otherwise unknown disturbances may arise, which can have a negative influence on the results.

Neurosurgical Ergonomics Paradigm 1. Each surgical procedure on a patient's brain first takes place in the surgeon's brain. This is a description of the operative procedure by means of neuropsychology. The surgeon's effectiveness and manual abilities are seen as a result of an action in his or her brain (Fig. 5.4):
- The surgeon's brain is the main surgical instrument.
- The use of the surgeon's brain defines the surgeon's art.
- The cortical representation defines the surgeon's skills.

For example, guidance of a surgical microscope by means of a mouth-operated switch is more productive than use of a head-mounted optical tract system or pupillary guidance. This is because the eye-guided procedure or the head-guided procedure involves and interacts directly with motor perception of the rest of the body and this functional convergence, being difficult, adds irritation, thus making it difficult to break through this functional dissociation. On the other hand, the jaw musculature, which is not associated with the motor perceptions of the body, can take over the task of controlling an instrument without causing any problems of interaction. This is a natural

5

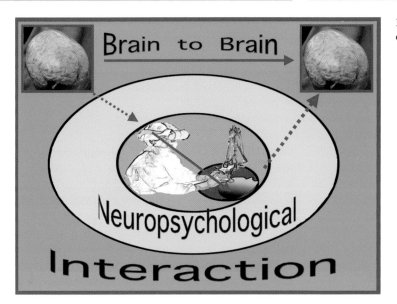

Fig. 5.4. Paradigm 1 for neurosurgical ergonomics: in the surgeon's brain

and extensive functional dissociation. Theoretically, these connections can be learned and practiced, but only with high-level financial investment, so that acceptance is poor.

The more accurately the human–system interface based on neuropsychological criteria is configured, the more successful the technical system will be. A good model is seen in the development of the computer mouse (see Fig. 5.8). The complicated cursor-guided tour with the keyboard has been replaced through incorporation of highly precise hand–eye coordination, and the outcome is excellent. The application of neuropsychological criteria has transformed the computer–human interface, since technical conversion of intelligent interfaces based on such criteria has thus been ergonomically realized.

Adequate Technical and Mental Ergonomics. Ergonomics is rarely considered in neurosurgery, and if it is the deliberations are mostly related to a detailed problem (Al-Mefty 1989; Nunez and Kaufman 1988; Perneczky et al. 1999; Yasargil et al. 1969). Current developments in neurosurgery are aimed at minimizing the entire trauma, including the additional trauma of implementing state-of-the-art techniques (Perneczky 1992; Perneczky and Fries 1998; M. Scholz et al. 2004). Simultaneously, the technical environment is also developing, with its own influence on this process.

As a result, the neurosurgeon has a large variety of systems, instruments, and computers to choose from, many of which are not 'compatible' with each other, few are advanced, and many are not adapted to the neurosurgeon's needs (Resch 1999). Design solutions are not adequate, as already reported elsewhere. It is

of critical importance to the effectiveness of these design resolutions that the entire development should have a primary goal; the ergonomic relationship between the operator and patient should not be affected (Al-Mefty 1989; Patkin 1977, 1981). The current generation of neuronavigation systems and intraoperative MRI and CT cause temporal, spatial, and ergonomic obstruction. It does, then, seem necessary to introduce the term 'ergonomic trauma' (Fig. 5.5).

In past years, the rapid technical development in neurosurgery has become a very problematic subject owing to an accumulation of disturbing factors, which must be recognized:

On the one hand, new equipment is being developed too fast, insofar as decisions on a technical system turn out months later to be wrong. On the other hand, development is characterized less and less by the tendency for the equipment to be integrated into the entire spatial circumstances of the operating room and the daily routine there. The ergonomics are just disregarded! The result, understandably, is ergonomic and chronological 'trauma' to the patients (Resch 1999; see also, for example, Steinmeier et al. 1998; Tronnier et al. 1999; Wirtz and Kunze1998). Nonetheless, there are still attempts to ignore these important relationships in study design (Paleologos et al. 2000);however, these problems are well known and have already been the subject of some discussion (Chandler 2000; Kelly 2000; Maciunas 2000; Shekar 2000).

The introduction of 'neuroimaging' and its basic computer-assisted planning system has led to increasingly precise anatomical diagnosis and operational design. These specialized systems help in the implementation of these precise procedures; so-

Fig. 5.5. Cerebral cybernetics: man /
environment

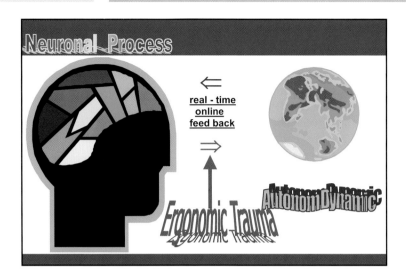

called neuronavigation systems, which compensate for the lacking real-time pattern of the navigational systems; and 'intraoperative imaging' (CT, MRI), accompanied by 'functional imaging' and 'intraoperative monitoring.' These new developments have resulted in degradation of functional ergonomics, which has apparently gone unnoticed, since the technology this would have required was not yet fully developed. Titles such as "*Interactive Image-Guided Neurosurgery*" (Maciunas 1993) or "*Neurosurgery for the Millenium*" (Apuzzo 1992) did not just provide valuable stimuli to the technical evolution potential of the future, but also implied some technical 'euphoria.' Nonetheless, the 'art' of neurosurgical technology is mutating and the ergonomic problems are simply being ignored.

All ergonomic mistakes result in a loss of quality and in wear and tear. The instruments must be constructed in such a way as to allow the hands to work in a relaxed way, without hindering the approach. Every handpiece is extra-axial to a thin, pipe-shaped, functional piece. The monitor should be at just the same height as the operator's head and so sited that it can be seen by a direct look across the thorax of the patient. A better alternative is an LCD display or an HMD system. The other devices should be in comfortable reach of the outstretched hand. The endoscope fixture must be positioned precisely and so that no expenditure of energy such as is needed for the microscope is required, and it must be able to hold every position with no oscillation. The optical set-up of the endoscope must be adaptable and variable to suit the way the instruments have to be prepared.

Paraendoscopic video preparation through a burr hole or keyhole is completely different from microsurgical preparations in the ergonomics concerning posture, line of vision, and manipulation methods. In our special laboratory setting, which is rather close to life surgery but still far removed from the stress of real-life surgery, the absolute correlation between the ergonomics of the setting and instruments and the results, or even the chance of get any result at all, is quite evident. In the final analysis, the resulting factor is the perfect cooperation of all these factors, including, and even in particular, the actual operator. This interaction is the *overall-ergonomics*.

The ability to work under these ergonomically acceptable conditions requires a specialized training, because the course of this laboratory work is becoming more intense, so that further developments of this method can make more rapid results and new experiences possible. However, problems will become more dominant, as safety problems in clinical application of the method show. This '*problem profile*' is a result of the laboratory work and is simultaneously also a *development profile* for further developments. In this connection, we may find that the training capabilities reach a reasonable level because at least in the development phase the decisive question is whether the technology should be adapted to the operating surgeon, or vice versa. In everyday clinical operating, the surgeon does not have any choice; but during the laboratory work it was decided that the technician must compensate when too many or too difficult technical and ergonomic problems whose end-effect could potentially be a clinical disaster arise in conditions not characterized by any harmful factors. Therefore, the description of such results is relevant. Logically it is not our goal to improve the training for compensation of technical failures, but urgent necessities are:

- Picture screen quality – as the results of the laboratory work prove, the *resolution of a subarachnoid trabecula* should be made visible.
- The *endoscope* needs a *zoom feature* to compensate for the *endoscopic-instrument competition* problem, so that the endoscope for the instrument, if required, can make more space (it can be pulled back) without any decrease in the optical quality.
- The *endoscopic fixture* is one of the determining safety factors through appropriate ergonomics with the para-endoscopic technique.
- During an operation only an inadequate minimum number of microsurgical instruments can be used, because more simply do not fit through a burr hole. The *instruments* must belong to a very *new instrument family*, because they are intended to allow secure priming for para-endoscopic and coaxial procedures. Therefore, all instruments must have a *borehole-adaptable design*.
- With the combined training, when clinical necessity dictates the use of such *devices, transendoscopic ultrasound* with *online analysis and navigation* and the *holmium–YAG laser* for *non-mechani-cal preparation* can both be integrated without much effort. Further devices must be tested, such as the transendoscopic ultrasound aspirator, intraoperative mini-MR, and the transendoscopic aneurysm clip.

In summary, it can be seen from experience in practical laboratory work that para-endoscopic morphological results were made possible only by *ergonomic changes* to the entire process. Furthermore, in the near future the question will not apply to the techniques currently available in clinical practice and used hitherto, and not because the absence of detailed developments means they are *not sufficiently secure* for clinical implementation in para-endoscopic surgery; more importantly it will pertain to the fact that they do not take sufficient account of the importance of the *ergonomics being suitable for daily clini*cal use.

It has been shown that in their present form most instruments and devices cause problems with the *ergonomics* of the system 'preparation technician–preparation object' (head) (ergonomic trauma; see Resch 1999) and cannot be smoothly integrated into the existing process except, on an individual basis and at the expense of safety and efficiency. Some compensation through training during the laboratory work has in fact proved possible, but does not

seem to be a reasonable goal of further developments (Resch 2002).

Ergonomic Trauma and Ergonomic Zones

The problem of ergonomics has various effects in different localizations within the operating room. It is possible to define various 'ergonomic zones.'
1. Surgeon's hands and patient's head
2. Surgeon's body and patient's head
3. Operative setting
4. Operation suite

Neurosurgical Ergonomics Paradigm 2. The operative environment can be described with reference to *gestalt* theory (Fig. 5.6).
- The operative environment has a meaningful structure of virtual emerging orbits.
- The ergonomic sensitivity of each orbit is different.
- The degree to which disturbances affect a procedure increases with increasing ergonomic sensitivity.

A catalog of these disturbances shows how diverse and complex the processes are from a neuropsychological viewpoint and how they take a radical effect:
1. The *video hand–eye-coordination* is much poorer than the microscope hand–eye coordination
2. The problematic fact of a narrow entrance (borehole) means that mainly *coaxial manipulation* of the instruments is possible.
3. The endoscope travels to the anatomical region concerned; therefore the visualization is intracranial. The endoscope performs in a similar way to a microsurgical instrument, so that *moving images* are used for *navigation*, which is very disconcerting at first and repeatedly leads to difficulties.
4. Since the endoscope and the instruments arrive at the 'entrance' with equal 'rights to space,' this introduces competition between the *endoscope and the instruments*, which can occasionally become dangerously puzzling when the picture no longer matches in with what is felt when they are moved by hand, so that *endoscope-instrument coordination* must be mastered.
5. Since there is always a blind field without visual instrument control behind the lens, and even next to the lens there is always a blind angle, which is different for every endoscope, a *para-endoscopic guided* tour must be learned; although endoscopically controlled introduction of the instruments is preferred as the safer method, in difficult cases

Fig. 5.6. Paradigm 2 for neurosurgical ergonomics: ergonomic zones

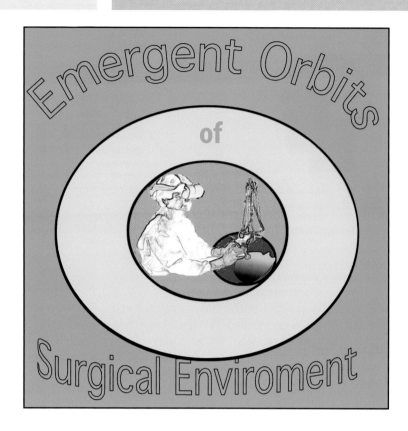

Fig. 5.7. Ergonomic zones and ergonomic trauma

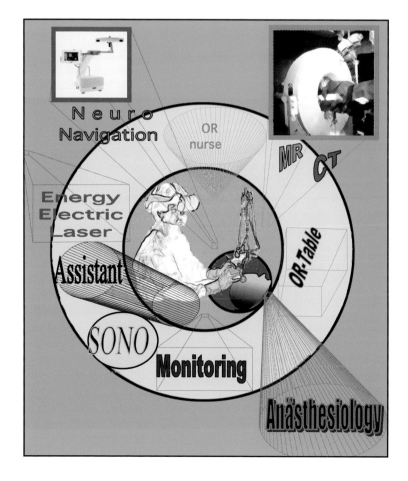

5

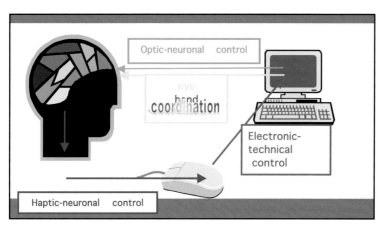

Fig. 5.8. Cybernetics of intuitive control: example computer–mouse

this is not always easily done, particularly if there are two instruments to be controlled.

6. The optical qualities of the endoscope lead to a *3-D effect* that is only virtual. This results in a '*fish-eye*' effect, which distorts the geometry of the image.

   This means there is no possibility of estimating *distance* and *size* correctly. Therefore a new *optical–visual perception* must be created.

7. A problem already known from the microsurgical techniques persists in an intensified form: the image seen shows only a part of the anatomy. The biggest part of the *anatomical mosaic* is present only in the mind. This problem is intensified considerably when a para-endoscopic preparation is used, so that a high level of *mental neuronavigational ability* must be applied (Fig. 5.7).

The ergonomic zones extend from the center of the surgeon's hands to the patient's head. This is the 'red zone,' in which ergonomically problematic mistakes have an intense effect. Three further zones have been defined (orange, yellow, green), all of which are sensitive to ergonomic disturbances. Some functional units in the operating room affect several zones. Devices that affect several zones obviously involve a higher ergonomic risk. You must, for example, be 'red zone adaptable' even when you are working predominantly in the green zone.

The ergonomic zone model shows the developer how the product needs to adapt to a given setting and be amenable to integration. New technical achievements should be measured by the ergonomic problems they cause. A robot that carries out a simple biopsy, for example, is ten times as expensive as a neurosurgeon and works at only one fifth the speed of a neurosurgeon: the robot can do nothing else, and is effectively an ergonomic catastrophe, even though in a single dimension it is more precise (Fig. 5.12).

Intuitive Operability

The most important goal involving the application of ergonomics to a neuropsychologically appropriate configuration of the human–machine interface intuitive operability of the system. This takes a cybernetic with both real-time and online feedback mechanisms. The cybernetic model 'computer mouse,' for example, has the following intelligent interfaces:

Configuration: The natural closed-loop control system (real-time/online feedback), the eye–hand coordination (blue/yellow), is extended to an open-loop control system, the eye–hand–mouse–display coordination (Fig. 5.8; blue–red–green). The configuration of the interfaces is such that the computer is integrated into the closed-loop control system. The special feature in this theory that leads to an intelligent solution is finding the 'black box,' which is in the brain (colored). The neuropsychological knowledge counts on the fact that the brain identifies the entire course of events of the mouse–cursor operation as a neurological process and accompanies it in real time. This neuropsychological subordination concerning the black box makes this closed-loop control system the definitive one (Fig. 5.8).

It is essential that the demand for a real-time/online characteristic be met to allow a technical system to be integrated into a neurological closed-loop control system and, consequently, intuitive operability to be achieved.

Therefore, many so-called neuronavigation systems can be excluded, since they only impersonate navigation. Every shift in the brain ruins the navigation because the data outcome is wrong. Only intraoperative imaging can achieve this navigation, and then only when the real-time and online mechanisms work, which makes CT and MR systems ineffective.

The remaining techniques are:
- Direct visual techniques, such as microscopy and endoscopy
- X-Ray (high exposure to radiation; used as 'scout' technique)
- Intraoperative sonography
- Mini-MR system

Neuronavigation, robotics, and virtual reality do not have any reasonable contribution to a system in which the human capabilities remain more direct and economical and can be successfully integrated. This changes immediately in areas where this integration is impossible, such as in the case of space travel, and in high-risk areas.

Intuitive operability relies on:
- Real-time function
- Online function
- Integrated, multimodulated interface
- Integration in a neurohaptically controlled loop system
- Ergonomic realization
- Synchronization and convergence of all interactive coordinate systems into a single interactive coordinate system
- Direction of the coordination system into the navigator

Where Should the Interactive Coordination System Be Localized? This is a key question for intuitive operation. In fact, there are many coordinate systems in the operating room that can be influenced by the operating surgeon. For example, every image archive system has its own coordinates. The human being has a coordinate system in every joint, all of which are integrated into the body pattern. The technical coordinate systems must be synchronized and made to converge for an intuitive contact to be achieved. All coordinate systems must be aligned with each other and also aligned primarily with the patient's head. The imaging can only be displayed on one system. To ensure that the external coordinates of the imaging do not limit the intrinsic dynamics of the operating surgeon the use of an HMD system is ideal.

With the current developments, the coordinate system, an orthogonal, mathematical system, is created in the head of the patient through imaging (CT/MRI) and with navigational techniques. All this, however, means that the operating surgeon is given a mathematical area in advance, which intuitive navigation excludes for the following reasons:
- Lacking real-time function
- Lacking online function
- Lacking emergence

It is possible to be guided by the coordinate system of the imaging (CT/MR) instead of by the operation, which means by the operator him-/herself. The surgery must be surgeon guided and not image guided!

The visual abilities of the operator are generally not used with contemporary systems, so that constant inspection of the system and continuous compensation of its weaknesses are needed. This disturbs the operation process far more than is obvious. Should lack of talent and experience also be eliminated, this too could lead to unforeseeable consequences for the patient. Therefore, patients should be introduced to the term 'ergonomic trauma' (Resch 1999).

For the aforementioned systems with real-time and online functions to be intuitively operable it must be possible for the operating surgeon's entry into the working environment to go smoothly. This is necessary so that s/he can receive the data needed. Today's systems supply only intellectually controllable and one-dimensional data (Fig. 5.9).

Synchronization and convergence of the coordinate systems do not solve the problem of how operation is achieved intuitively. The solution can be found by means of two strategies:
- With mathematical coordinates
- With biological coordinates

5

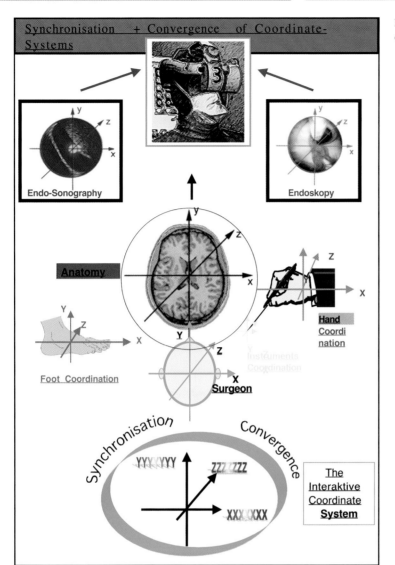

Fig. 5.9. Synchronization and convergence of coordinate system

With Mathematical Coordinates. After synchronization and convergence, it is necessary to decide where the controlled convergence and synchronization of the coordinate system must be localized. At present, directing the active coordinates toward the inside of the patient's head prevents intuitive operation. The technical model used to illustrate this is that of the combat jet: in this case the leading coordinate system is not directed into the target area but into the navigator itself (Fig. 5.10).

With Biological Coordinates. Conventionally, the products of optical and analogous systems are referred to as 'visualization' and those of digital systems, as 'imaging.' The capability of the human eye differs dramatically from the imaging capability of a computer. Weizaecker (1950) expressed this in his book "*Der Gestaltkreis*": "*The visual apparatus in-cluding the CNS does not have any mathematical ideas of spatial capability; rather, it reconstructs itself each time*" (Weizaecker 1950). A digital media separates the task description and the hardware for its execution, while both were optimized inseparably in the course of evolution in the brain; there is an original context (Poggio 1987). Thus, attempts to teach computers the ability of sight have shown that sight is a highly complex information-processing process (Cooper and Shepard 1987; Gelding 1987; Gillam 1987; Regan et al. 1987; Roth 1999). Neurobiologists consider sight to be a learned process of recognition, and also a neural/microevolutionary process of enormous speed, which many have referred to as a 'sense' (Edelmann 1992).

In conclusion, it must be emphasized that the visual grammar (Gregory 1974; Sacks 1992) is completely separate from the digital, mathematical rules, be-

Fig. 5.10. Mathematical coordinates within the navigator. The best-known model of using mathematical coordinates for navigation is the jet. The synchronized and converged coordinates of the jet, the target, and the monitor are linked to a single active and intuitively maneuverable coordinate system, i.e., the pilot's joystick. Only this enables the pilot to aim at the target at high speed

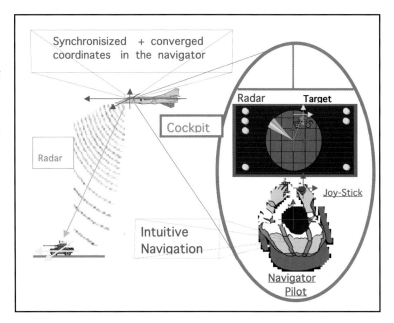

Fig. 5.11. Biological coordinates within the navigator

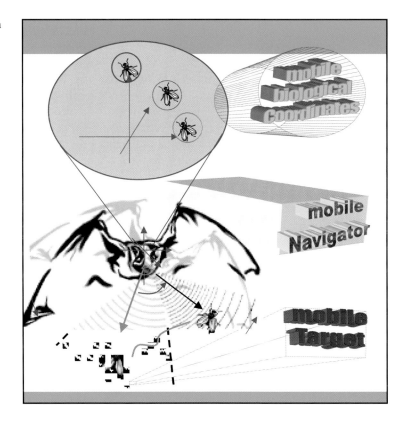

cause its level of complexity will never be achieved by digital media (Sacks 1989a, b).

We must therefore consider what importance attaches to visualization and imaging and explore the individual importance of each; on the basis of the known higher competence and high reliability of visualization, this appears to be the more important. The current technical evolution in neurosurgery does not seem to be affected by these connections, and evaluation of the current technical developments seems to be giving rise to minimal optimism. The term-artifact 'technology' is therefore illusory, because current developments do not justify use of the particle 'logos' (Resch et al. 1997a–c; Urban and Hasenbrink 1995).

5

Digital imaging systems are based on a Cartesian coordinate system and evolve in a pixel or voxel world. Visualization, however, for example during a brain operation, uses biological coordinates, which is what distinguishes it from the differences described above.

Biological coordinates facilitate intuitive navigation because the structures visualized with the coordinates are identical. The identification is made by structural analysis and not through numbers. Biological coordinates are normally already synchronized, converged, interactive, and localized in the navigator. The brain of the operating surgeon is optimized through biological coordinates, so that the entire mental potential can be exploited by the navigator.

This depends on shaping the process of developments through proper decisions, and not leaving it to chance.

The bat and the dolphin are optimal biological models (Fig. 5.11).

Interactive Operability

Intuitive operability does not mean that the operating surgeon can make modifications. 'Intuitive operation' of the system implies that intervention in the system is possible. This leads to a variety of interaction, i.e., *interactive operability*. If a mental problem is presented the interactive operability displays a technical problem.

The space of *emergence* is also achieved without VR techniques, because the immersive qualities are produced directly through intelligent interfaces with the actual space and not through a virtual copy. The actual illustration is produced through visualization techniques or, less frequently, imaging techniques when they have real-time and online qualities. In the same way, the presence of the operating surgeon is part of the system, as is the use of the actual space. The detour required when a VR image is used is not necessary and not beneficial; in the end-effect, it is actually detrimental. This detriment does not become obvious until the operator is not present (danger zones, space, remote location, etc.).

Two development strategies are currently in use to achieve intuitive and interactive operability:
- Virtual reality (VR) techniques
- Intelligent human–machine-interfaces with consistent ergonomically flexibility

VR technique. The overriding advantage of the VR technique is that it allows emergency rooms with immersing qualities. Therefore, the user can enter the space interactively. High-density data are presented to him/her as transposed experiences.

This technique is still beset by teething troubles, however, because the technical conversion of neuropsychological capabilities of the human brain can hardly be achieved. Investigation of these abilities is still in the very early stages.

The main drawbacks of VR techniques are related to their vital importance in the crucial considerations below, which are presented in greater detail.

Modern Imaging and Virtual Reality. The main problem in modern imaging lies in recognizing the boundaries of its competence. It is a problem both for the theoretical evolution of evolution and for its scientific nature that experience has frequently led to confusion of the use of state-of-the-art techniques, e.g., VR techniques, with scientific experiments. Marcuse described this oddity as along ago as in 1964, at a sociological level: "*In turn we face one of the most agitated aspects of the advanced industrial civilization: the rational character of their irrationality.*"

Like 'technology,' 'virtual reality' is a word artifact: a word case that is contradictory in a treacherous way. The virtuality is not, however, a technical finding, but appertains to the anatomy and physiology of the process that is called consciousness (Edelmann 1992). Virtual reality is historically regarded as a product of the military industry, and given its original aim the etymological birth defects should not come as any surprise. With VR, the above problem of the assessment of competence is a sociopsychological dimension that cannot be easily estimated. Such statements as: "*We still know very little about the psychological influence that interactive computer media has on its users*" and, '*One question that needs to be examined is to what degree the "Virtual World" will take the place of other forms of interpersonal relationships and communication*' give some indication of what the future holds (Schroeder 2001).

The main advantage of VR is that it is noninvasive and is a multimodal information experience within a confined environment, which enables the human brain to integrate information in a conscious form (Edelmann 1992; Resch et al. 1997b). It is burdened, however, by a dangerous disadvantage insofar as the fascination of this presentation is rationally difficult to control, because it has an effect analogous to that of advertising spots. We should not wonder, then, why so many specialists fall into a trap when it comes to the critical question of competence. It is difficult to discriminate between actual illustrated competence and the simulated competence of interactive media, because the attractiveness of the presentation is not rationally analyzed but is rather focused on the sublibic functions. Suppose, for example, that a computer-generated virtual trip through the ventricle system fascinates an experienced neurosurgeon, who then has hardly any capacity free and does not have an adequate picture library of mental images against which s/he can test his/her virtual trip of competence. The displacement of the angiographic architecture of the brain through CT and MR leaves obvious gaps in the cerebral bookshelves of neurosurgery, which are already becoming manifest in everyday life. Giannotta's hope that these gaps can be compensated by computers and robotics is almost a little naive). Whether there is a chance that digital techniques can replace solid scientific judgment and infralimbic effects (and irrational reasons that we will not go into here), with an injection of scientific methods and methodology in exchange, is something that all those involved will have to decide. Levy (1998)surely had good reasons for the extraordinary comment he made on Auer and Auer's work, "*Virtual Endoscopy for Planning and Simulation of Minimally Invasive Neurosurgery*" (Auer and Auer 1998), on which his final word was: "*We recommend that processing be performed by a team that includes neurosurgeons and neuroradiologists*" (Resch et al. 1997a,b).

The more we know about the functions of the human brain, the more critical it is to evaluate the current digital media breakdowns. Human brains, including those of neurosurgeons, can fall victim to unreal digital data, because our brain is has not yet evolved to its optimal stage. If we were to eliminate the need for solving problems that do not present themselves, such as how to practice the imitation of reality through imaging, we could concentrate on a productive and exclusively parallel function of the VR: supply of an assessment of a real visualization with an eccentric orientation model. The visualization is the pedestrian going through the streets of a city; VR is the city map, with capabilities of interaction and anticipation. The pedestrian decides whether to cross the street, with reference to the city map in his hand but always with his or her eyes on the street (Resch 2003).

Intelligent Human–Machine Interfaces with Consistent Ergonomic Realization

Unlike the VR technique, this strategy exists today, and offers the reassurance of greater safety and competence. Full exploitation of ergonomic conversion and the applications of intelligent interfaces already possible enable us to do presently without the VR technique. The intelligence, according to these criteria for developed projects, is embedded in the compatibility of the individual components and in their maximal simplification. The combination of all these aspects increases the acceptance considerably. This simplification is successful because we are refraining from any attempt at technical imitation of the human capabilities of the operator. On the contrary, the operator inputs these capabilities as a part of the system. Therefore, the education and training of the operator are again very important. This project relies on the fact that training takes place in any case and is cheaper than the more expensive and complicated 'technical expert systems' that hardly deliver what they promise.

Precision Integrated with Complexity (Fig. 5.12)

As in the case of neuronavigation and of robots, people will cite the 'precision' rating in arguments, but use it to mean one-dimensional mathematical precision. Sometimes the term 'operative precision' is used in critical papers, which is more helpful as this comes

Fig. 5.12. Point where complexity and precision cross

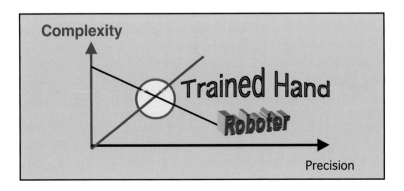

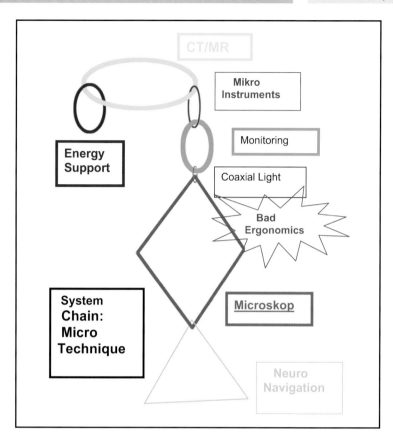

Fig. 5.13. System chain: microtechnique

closer to the actual situation and mostly involves inaccuracy that is greater by a factor of up to 10 than the technical precision value.

What is not often mentioned is that the special feature of the human hand, which should be seen as the main factor in all this, is the combination of precision and complexity. Only the functional maneuvers of the hand make anything possible. As always in biology, we can start with the human hand as the ideal interface between precision and complexity.

Microtechnique ⇒ Microsystem Technique (Miniaturization)

In every functional chain the weakest link determines the result. It is therefore essential to develop the entire sequence of equipment to give a system with uniform quality and the same functional direction (Fig. 5.13).

The microtechnique already in use in some cases must be developed into a microsystem technique. Continuous development of the microtechnique to create a microsystem technique will result in the functional chain's being harmonized and reshaped ergonomically (Fig. 5.14).

The greatest importance attaches to:
- Miniaturization
- Simplification
- Integration of single components
- Modular system
- Adaptation to ergonomic zones

Neurosurgical Ergonomics Paradigm 3. The operative procedure is a chaotic system. This means the operation is described by fuzzy logic (Fig. 5.15):
- A chaotic system shows exactly defined parameters, but its outcome is never predictable.
- A chaotic system can only be influenced by its peripheral parameters. Some of the peripheral parameters of an operation are:
  - Equipment and design (technique)
  - Physical fitness of the surgeon (body)
  - Mental fitness of the surgeon (mind)
  - Cooperation of the team members (interpersonal interaction)

Fig. 5.14. System chain: microsystem technique

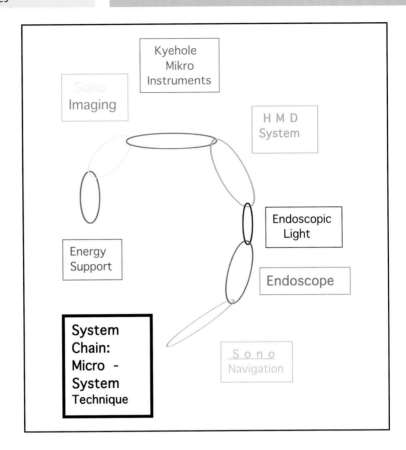

Fig. 5.15. Paradigm 3 for neurosurgical ergonomics: fuzzy logic

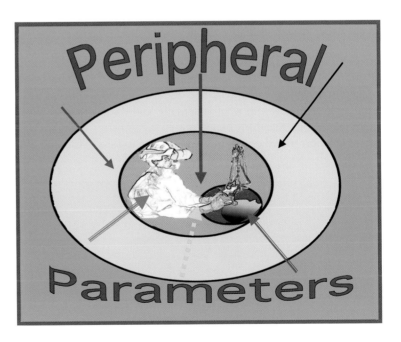

Essential changes to achieve a harmonious functional chain are:

- Replacing the microscope with the endoscope
- Replacing the monitor with an HMD system with multidimensional imaging
- Integration of the support in the endoscope bracket
- Intraoperative imaging with sonography
- Navigation interface for sonography as an auxiliary interpretation system
- Borehole-efficient 'knitting needle' instruments

Final Reflections

This chapter on future concepts in minimally invasive neurosurgery seems rather theoretical in a book dealing with a neurosurgical imaging tool. However, in the author's experience only a good balance between technical and intellectual equipment can provide for an evolution that is not beset by uncontrollable dangers (Fig. 5.16a).

ENS is understood within an environment of ergonomic evolution of the whole process in the operating room. It is part of the minimally invasive concept of the future: para-endoscopic intuitive computer-assisted operation-system (Fig. 5.16b). That means that the ergonomic system, the microhabitat, is not made up just of the technical equipment, but also of the patient and, especially, the surgeon. The major blind spot of neurosurgeons is their own brains (Paradigm 1: "Neuropsychological Interaction"). Consequently, technical equipment and today's mental training are at odds with what is actually known of neuropsychology. An athlete being trained to compete for an Olympic medal or a pilot being trained to fulfill a military purpose is mentally better prepared for his or her task than neurosurgeons usually are when faced with a human brain in trouble.

The neurosurgeon's brain is a high-potential VR (narrative) system. The most intense connections involving the brain are not those with the environment or the body it is housed in, but those that take place within it self. Each VR technique should be seen as in competition with the human brain in training efforts. It does not seem prudent to neglect this capacity of the human brain and to invest indolently in technical solutions only.

The understanding of ENS imaging and visualization, as of imaging in general, depends on the size of the anatomical image library in the surgeon's brain and all the virtual surgical clips on which s/he can draw as s/he anticipates the procedure mentally. A technical tool that interrupts or disturbs the relation between the patient's brain and the surgeon's brain mentally or physically should have no future, as it handicaps the surgical art (Paradigm 2: "Ergonomic Zones"). ENS fits in smoothly with endoscopy and microsurgery, but from the microsystem point of view it is still not mature and needs to be better integrated in a single system.

It seems to give us a good, and perhaps necessary, feeling about ourselves if we can think that the surgical process is rational and completely controllable. However, this is not the case as far as the function of the surgeon's brain is concerned. It might be more helpful to view the surgical procedure as a 'chaotic system' that can be described by fuzzy logic. With this concept we will focus on the peripheral parameters that are the only links that have any influence on the outcome within such a chaotic system (Paradigm 3: "Chaotic System"). The author's qualitative experi-

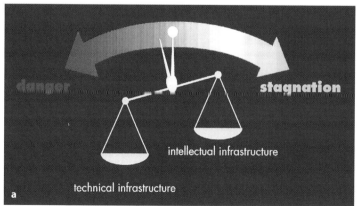
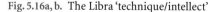
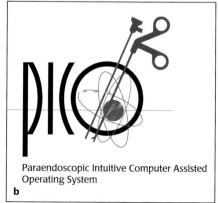

Paraendoscopic Intuitive Computer Assisted Operating System

Fig. 5.16a, b. The Libra 'technique/intellect'

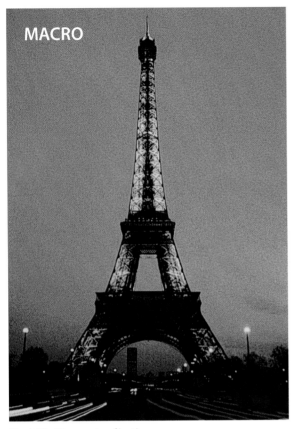

Fig. 5.17. Macro-visualization

ripheral parameters, which prevents any surgeon from performing at an optimum level. Such peripheral parameters are described by the three paradigms of ergonomics in neurosurgery. The future focus in the evolution of minimally invasive neurosurgery must be the synergistic mechanism and interdependence of all three paradigms; if one is disregarded the others cannot be fulfilled.

We have progressed through three major stages of visualization in neurosurgery as far as technical tools are concerned: macro-, micro-, and endovisualization. We can symbolize this by illustrations of a well-known building visualized in each of these different ways (Figs. 5.17, 5.18, 5.19, respectively). Each visualization has its own specific implications for ergonomics, which affect the entire procedure and all the manual and mental abilities necessary for success.

The last step in technical change in viewing is a completely different dimension from the three mentioned and illustrated above. We change from visualization to imaging. The ergonomic implications of this 'virtual' imaging (Fig. 5.20) are still not clear, as the mental and neuropsychological effects are not sufficiently well understood to allow us to estimate all the effects on both the surgeon and the procedure.

This paradigmatic journey is presented as a series of technical steps, but the same evolution can be viewed with an historical perspective.

Since the time of Leonardo da Vinci the word 'imago' has come to mean something quite different from our 'image,' and even more different from 'imaging.' Da Vinci did not believe in citations, but tended to translate earlier sentences into sayings that fitted better in his own time. Today he would probably no longer say, "*To see is to understand,*" perhaps prefer-

ence in 25 years of laboratory work and his study of neurosurgeons over a long period (one series of very eminent neurosurgeons and one of 'standard' neurosurgeons) has led to the hypothesis that the outcome can best be influenced by controlling the peripheral parameters in advance. Too much concentration and energy is lost in trying to control badly prepared pe-

Fig. 5.18. Micro-visualization

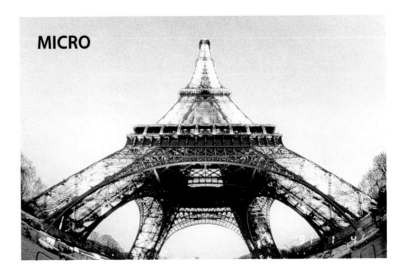

5

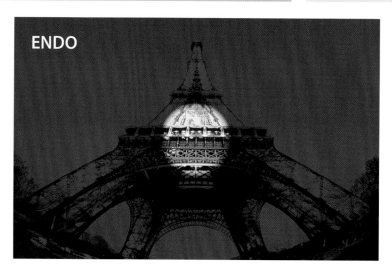

Fig. 5.19. Endo-visualization

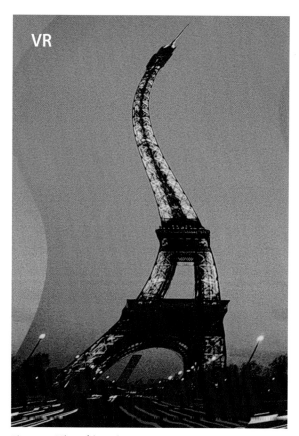

Fig. 5.20. Virtual imaging

ring, "It's not possible to understand everything we can see." Da Vinci's pictures have never been nothing but images; rather, he always understood them as symbols and concepts. His main vision in his art and his scientific work was directed at symbolizing the invisible.

Imaging is completely different, as it has no symbolic characteristic; there is no 'message' in an imaging. Moreover, imaging has lost the intuitive context for the spectator, while da Vinci produced his pictures with his own hands and was conscious of each detail of technique and methodology and of how his pictures related to reality. Da Vinci had the ability to write with both brain hemispheres, and his pictures were writings from a neuropsychological point of view.

Imaging is made up mainly of information, and only a small part of the information present in an imaging is seen and used by neurosurgeons. The amount of imaging output does not increase the benefit, because it is limited by the ability of the spectator to manage all the imaging masses mentally. In addition, many images can make the brain blind to their meaning, even if there were any chance of understanding the real meaning of such complex artifacts as fMRT or PET, for example. Da Vinci created a concept-guided science and not an image-guided one, and we can assume that he would prefer to speak to us if he realized our blindness to the meaning of what we call an image and what we believe that imaging can mean in neurosurgery. He would realize that conceptuality and awareness of context are lacking in our technical images and would change from painting to writing to convey his ideas to us and make the invisibility of a message visible (Fig. 5.21).

Figure 5.21 is entitled „*The Vision of the Cat*," but it really has nothing to do with cats, rather symbolizing the relation between endoscopy and ultrasound in ENS. It is not an imaging but an 'imago,' and to see it is to understand it.

Fig. 5.21. The vision of the cat

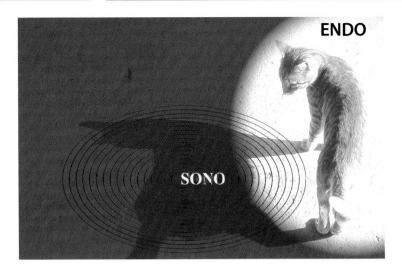

ENS imaging can only be understood if the images are seen in conceptual relation to anatomy, geometry, ultrasound physics, and operative imaging problems such as targeting and orientation.

In future, the emphasis will have to move away from image-guided and back to concept-guided neurosurgery if the masses of images are really to culminate in any benefit to our patients.

References

AIUM (1993) The bioeffect and safety of diagnostic ultrasound. American Institute of Ultrasound in Medicine and Biology, Rockville, Md

Albert FK, Wirtz C R, Tronnier VM et al (1998) Intraoperative diagnostic and interventional MRI in neurosurgery: first experience with an "open MR" sytem. In: Hellwig D, Bauer BL (eds) Minimally invasive techniques for neurosurgery. Springer, Berlin Heidelberg New York

Al-Mefty O (1989) Surgery of the cranial base. Kluwer Academic, Boston, pp 3-11

Apuzzo MLJ (1992) Neurosurgery for the Third Millenium. American Association of Neurological Surgeons, USA, pp 11-23

Apuzzo MLJ (1996) New dimension of neurosurgery in the realm of high technology: Possibilities, practicalities, realities. Neurosurgery 38:625-639

Aschermann M, Fergusson JJ (1992) Present possibilities of use of intravascular ultrasound examinations. Cas Lek Cesk 131(17):516-520

Aschermann M, Fergusson JJ, Raymond-Martimbeau P (1992) Endovascular echography. J Mal Vasc 17 Suppl B:123-126

Auer LM, Auer DP (1998) Virtual endoscopy for planning and simulation of minimally invasive neurosurgery. Neurosurgery 43(3):529-537; discussion 43:537-548

Auer LM, van Velthoven V (1990) Intraoperative ultrasound imaging in neurosurgery. Springer, Heidelberg Vienna New York

Auer LM, Holzer P, Ascher PW, Heppner F (1988) Endoscopic neurosurgery. Acta Neurochir (Wien) 90(1-2): 1-14

Black P, Mehta V (2000) Comment in: Wirtz CR, Knauth M, Staubert A et al (eds) Clinical evaluation and follow-up results for intraoperative magnetic resonance imaging in neurosurgery. Neurosurgery 46:1112-1120

Black PMcL, Moriarty T, Alexander E III et al (1997) Development and implementation of intraoperative magnetic resonance imaging and its neurosurgical application. Neurosurgery 41:831-845

Caemaert J, Abdullha J, Calliauw L et al (1992) Endoscopic treatment of suprasellar arachnoid cysts. Acta Neurochir (Wien) 119:68-73

Cappabianca P, Alfieri A, de Divitiis E (1998) Endoscopic endonasal transsphenoidal approacho the sella: Twards functional endoscopic pituitary surgery. Minim Invasive Neurosurg 41:66-73s

Cappabianca P, Alfieri A, Colao A et al (1999) Endoscopic endonasal transsphenoidal approach: an additional reason in support of surgery in the management of pituitary lesions. Skull Base Surg 9:109-116

Cavaye DM, Tabbara MR, Kopchok GE, Laas TE, White RA (1991) Three dimensional vascular ultrasound imaging. Am Surg 57:751-755

Chadduck WM (1989) Perioperative sonography. J Child Neurol 4 Suppl: S91-100

Chandler WF (2000) Comment. In: Paleologos TS, Wadley JP, Kitchen ND, Thomas GGT (2000) Clinical utility and cost-effectiveness of intracranial imageguided craniotomy: clinical comparision between conventional and image-guided meningeoma surgery. Neurosurgery 47:40-48

Cohen AR, Haines SJ (eds) (1995) Minimally invasive techniques in neurosurgery. Williams & Wilkins, Baltimore

Cooper LA, Shepard RN (1987) Rotation in der räumlichen Vorstellung. In Ritter M Wahrnehmung und visuelles System. Spektrum der Wissenschaft, Heidelberg, pp 122-131

Coy KM, Maurer G, Siegel RJ (1991) Intravascular ultrasound imaging: a current perspective. J Am Coll Cardiol 18(7):1811-1823

Cristante L (2000) A set of coaxial microsurgical instruments. Neurosurgery 45:1492-1494

Dagi TF (1997) Philosophical currents in the history of neurosurgery. In: Greenblatt SH (ed) A history of neurosurgery. American Association of Neurological Surgeons, USA, pp 561-578

Decq P (1998) Endoscopy in neurosurgery. Braun Druck, Tuttlingen

DEGUM (2001) Thermische Wirkung von Ultraschall. Ultraschall Med 22:105-106

Delcker A, Diener C (1994) Die quantitative Erfassung arteriosklerotischer Wandveränderungen der Karotiden mit einem dreidimensionalen Ultraschallverfahren. Akt Neurol 21:20-27

Docker MF, Duck FA (eds) (1991) The safe use of diagnostic ultrasound. British Medical Ultrasound Society/ British Institute of Radiology, London

Edelmann GM (1992) Göttliche Luft, vernichtendes Feuer. Wie der Geist im Gehirn entsteht. Piper, Munich, pp 19 359

EFSUMB, Pilling DW (2003) Diagnostic ultrasound exposure. EFSUMB Newslett 2003

Fahlbusch R, Nimsky C (2000) Comment. In: Wirtz CR, Knauth M, Staubert A et al (2000) Clinical evaluation and follow-up results for intraoperative magnetic resonance imaging in neurosurgery. Neurosurgery 46:1112-1120

Frank N, Grieshammer G , Zimmermann W (1994) A new miniature ultrasonic probe for gastrointestinal scanning: feasibility and preliminary results. Endoscopy 26(7):603-608

Fowlkes JB, Holland CK (2000) Mechanical bioeffects from diagnostic ultrasound: AIUM consensus statements. American Institute of Ultrasound in Medicine. J Ultrasound Med 219:69-72

Frank N, Holzapfel P, Wenk A (1994) Experience with a new endosonographic mini probe. Endoskopie Heute 3:238-244

Froelich J, Bien S, Hoppe M, Eggers F, Klose KJ (1996) An intracerebral sonographic catheter as an adjunct to stereotactic guided endoscopic procedue. Minim Invasive Neurosurg 39:9

Fukuhara T, Voster S J, Luciano M G (2000) Risk factors for failure of endoscopic third ventriculostomy for obstructive hydrocephalus. Neurosurgery 46:1100-1111

Fukushima T (1978) Endoscopic biopsy of intraventricular tumors with the use of ventriculofiberscope. Neurosurgery 2:110-113

Galloway RL, Berger MS, Bass WA, Maciunas RJ (1993) Registered intraoperative information: electrophysiology, ultrasound and endoscopy. In: Maciunas RJ (ed) Interactive image-guided neurosurgery. American Association of Neurological Surgeons, USA, pp 247-158, USA

Gillam B (1987) Geometrisch-optische Täuschungen. In Ritter M (ed) Wahrnehmung und visuelles System. Spektrum der Wissenschaft, Heidelberg, pp 104-113

Grönemeyer DHW, Lufkin RB (eds) (2001) Open field magnetic resonance imaging. Springer, Heidelberg Berlin New York

Grönemeyer DHW, Seibel RMM, Schmidt A et al (1994) Safety by CT/EBT or MRI for endoscopic instrument guidance. Minim Invasive Ther 3: Suppl 1

Grumme T (ed) (2001) Neurochirurgie in Deutschland. Blackwell Wissenschaft, Berlin Vienna

Grunert P, Perneczky A, Resch KDM (1995) Endoscopic procedures through the foramen interventriculare of Monro under stereotactic conditions. Minim Invasive Neurosurg 38:1995

Handler M H, Abbott R, Lee M (1994) A near-fatal complication of endoscopic third ventriculostomy: case report. Neurosurgery 35:525-527

Hayashi N, Endo S, Kurimoto M et al (1993) functional image-guided neurosurgical simulation system using computerized three-dimensional graphics and diploe tracing. Neurosurgery 37 (4) [whole issue]

Hopf N, Resch KDM, Ringel K, Perneczky A (1998) Endoscopic management of intracranial arachnoid cysts. In Hellwig D, Bauer LB (eds) Minimally invasive techniques for neurosurgery. Springer, Berlin Heidelberg New York

Horwitz AE, Sorensen N (1990) Intraoperativer Ultraschall in der pädiatrischen Neurochirurgie. Rontgenblatter 43(5):220-223

Isner JM, Rosenfield K, Losordo DW et al (1990) Percutaneous intravascular US as adjunct to catheter-based interventions: preliminary experience in patients with peripheral vascular disease. Radiology 175(1):61-70

Jenne J (2001) Kavitation in biologischem Gewebe. Ultraschall Med 22:200-207

Jho H-D, Carrau R L (1997) Endoscopic endonasal transsphenoidal surgery: experience with 50 patients. J Neurosurg 87:44-51

Jho H-D, Carrau R L, Ko Y, Daly MA (1996) Endoscopic pituitary surgery: an early experience. Surg Neurol 47:213-223

Kanazawa I, Shiraishi K, Kamitani H, Sato J, Masuzawa H (1986) Intraoperative ultrasonography through a burr hole: clinical trial of ultrasound-guided stereotactic surgery. No Shinkei Geka 14 (3 Suppl):295-230

Kelly PJ (2000) Comment. In: Paleologos TS, Wadley JP, Kitchen ND, Thomas GGT (2000) Clinical utility and cost-effectiveness of intracranial image-guided craniotomy: clinical comparision between conventional and image-guided meningioma surgery. Neurosurgery 47:40-48

Kikinis R, Gleason L, Moriarty TM et al (1996) Computer-assisted interactive three-dimensional planning for neurosurgical procedures. Neurosurgery 38:640-651

Kikinis R, Black PM, Jolez FA (1998) Image guided surgery. Aachener Workshop on Navigierte Hirnchirurgie, Aachen, 4-5 September 1998, abstract book, p 4

Kobayashi S, Okudera H (2000) Comment: In: Wirtz CR, Knauth M, Staubert A, Bonsanto MM, Sator K, Kunze S, Tronnier VM (2000) Clinical evaluation and follow-up results for intraoperative magnetic resonance imaging in neurosurgery. Neurosurgery 46:1112-1120

Koch C (2001) Thermische Wirkung von Ultraschall. Ultraschall Med 22:146-152

Kockro R A, Serra L, Tseng-Tsai Y et al (1999) Neurosurgical planning and training in a virtual reality environment. 11th European Congress of Neurological Surgery, Copenhagen, 19-24 September 1999, abstract book, p 75

Kockro RA, Serra L, Tseng-Tsai Y et al (2000) Planning and simulation of neurosurgery in a virtual reality environment. Neurosurgery 46:118-137

Köstering B (1991) Endosonographie-technische Grundlagen und klinische Anwendung. In: Zimmermann W, Nitzsche H, Schentke U, Sessner H (eds) Grenzen und Möglichkeiten der Endoskopie. Sonographie in der Gastroenterologie. Dresdener Kongreßbericht, vol 2. Dustri, Dresden

Koivukangas J, Louhisalmi Y, Alakuijala J, Oikarinen J (1993) Ultrasound-controlled neuronavigator-guided brain surgery. J Neurosurg. 79(1):36-42

Kuhn TS (1988) Die Struktur wissenschaftlicher Revolutionen, 8th edn. Surkamp, Frankfurt/Main

Kulkarni AV, Drake JM, Armstrong DC, Dirks PB (2000) Imaging correlates of endoscopic third ventriculostomy. J Neurosurg 92:915-919

Levy ML (1998) Virtual endoscopic simulations in neurosurgery: technical considerations and methodology (special editoral comment). Neurosurgery 43:538-548

Linke DB (1993) Hirnverpflanzung. Die erste Unsterblichkeit auf Erden. Rowohlt, Reinbek near Hamburg, pp 11-309

Linke DB (1997) Cognitive neuroscience foundations for a theory of neuronavigation. Computer-aided surgery: abstracts from CIS 97, pp 03-016

Linke DB (1999) Das Gehirn. CH Beck Wissen, Munich, pp 7-36

Lowry DW, Lowry DLB, Berga SL, Adelsen PD, Roberts MM (1996) Secondary amenorrhea due to hydrocephalus treated with endoscopic ventriculocisternostomy. J Neurosurg 85:1148-1152

Ludwig M, Wetzig H, Sauer A, Vetter H (1995) Experiences with use of an intravascular 6 French endosonography catheter in vivo. Klin Wochenschr 68(11):570-575

Maciunas RJ (ed) (1993) Interactive image-guided neurosurgery. American Association of Neurological Surgeons Publication Committee, USA

Maciunas RJ (2000) Comment. In: Paleologos TS, Wadley JP, Kitchen ND, Thomas GGT (2000) Clinical utility and cost-effectiveness of intracranial image-guided craniotomy: clinical comparison between conventional and image-guided meningioma surgery. Neurosurgery 47:40-48

McDonald JM (1993) Mental readiness and its link to performance excellence in surgery. Kinetek, Ottawa

McLaughlin MR, Wahlig JB, Kaufmann AM, Albright AL (1997) Traumatic basilar aneurysm after endoscopic third ventriculostomy. Case report. Neurosurgery 41:1400-1404

Makuuchi M, Torzilli G, Machi J (1998) History of intraoperative ultrasound. Ultrasound Med Biol 24(9):1229-1242

Manwaring KH, Krone KR (1992) Neuroendoscopy, vol 1. Mary Ann Liebert, New York

Masuzawa H, Kanazawa I, Kamitani H, Sato J (1985) Intraoperative ultrasonography through a burr-hole. Acta Neurochir (Wien) 77(1-2):41-45

Mayfrank L, Bertalanffy H, Spetzger U, Klein HM, Gilsbach JM (1994) Ultrasound-guided craniotomy for minimally invasive exposure of cerebral convexity lesions. Acta Neurochir (Wien) 131(3-4):270-273

Mintz GS, Pichard AD, Satler LF, Popma JJ, Kent KM, Leon MB (1993) Three-dimensional intravascular ultrasonography: reconstruction of endovascular stents in vitro and in vivo. J Clin Ultrasound 21(9):609-615

Moringlane JR , Voges M (1995) Real-time ultrasound imaging of cerebral lesions during „target point" stereotactic procedures through a burr hole (technical note). Acta Neurochir (Wien) 132(1-3):134-137

Müller S, Bartel T, Baumann G, Ebel R (1996) Preliminary report: Evaluation of three-dimensional echocardiographic volumetry by simultaneous thermal dilution in coronary heart disease. Cardiology 87:552-559

Neville RF, Bartorelli AL, Sidawy AN et al (1989) An in vivo feasibility study of intravascular ultrasound imaging. Am J Surg 158(2):142-145

Nunez G, Kaufman H (1988) Ergonomic considerations in the design of neurosurgery instruments. J Neurosurg 69: 436-441

Oi S, Samii A, Samii M (2005) Frameless free-hand maneuvering of a small-diameter rigid-rod neuroendoscope with a working channel used during high-resolution imaging. J neurosurg (Pediatrics 1) 102:113-118

Paleologos TS, Wadley JP, Kitchen ND, Thomas GGT (2000) Clinical utility and cost-effectiveness of intracranial image-guided craniotomy: clinical comparison between conventional and image-guided meningeoma surgery. Neurosurgery 47:40-48

Pandian NG, Sugeng L, Vogel M, Marx G (1993) Three-dimensional echocardiography: the future in cardiac imaging (highlights 6). Learning Center, Boston Mass

Patkin M (1977) Ergonomics applied to the practice of microsurgery. Aust NZ J Surg 47:320-328

Patkin M (1981) Ergonomics in microsurgery. Aust NZ J Obstet Gynaecol 21:134-136

Perneczky A (1992) Planning strategies for the suprasellar region. Philosophy of approaches. Neurosurgery 11: 343-348

Perneczky A, Fries G(1998) Endoscope-assisted brain surgery: evolution, basic concepts, and current technique. Neurosurgery 42:219-225

Perneczky A, Tschabitscher M, Resch KDM (1993) Endoscopic anatomy for neurosurgery (atlas/video). Thieme, Stuttgart

Perneczky A, Müller-Forell W, Lindert van E et al (1999) Keyhole concept in neurosurgery. Thieme, Stuttgart New York

Poggio T (1987) Wie Computer und Menschen sehen. In: Ritter M (ed) Wahrnehmung und visuelles System. Spektrum der Wissenschaft, Heidelberg, pp 78-89

Reddy K, Fewer H D, West M, Hill N C (1989) Slit ventricle syndrome with aqueduct stenosis: third ventriculostomy as a definitive treatment. Neurosurgery 23:756-759

Regan D, Beverly K, Cynader M (1987) Die Wahrnehmung von Bewegunen im Raum. In: Ritter M (ed) Wahrnehmung und visuelles System: Spektrum der Wissenschaft, Heidelberg, pp 90-103

Reich J, Onik GM, Maroon J (1988) Intracerebral biopsy hemorrhage: monitoring and intervention guided by intraoperative sonography. AJNR Am J Neuroradiol 9(6):1240-1241

Resch KDM (1999) MIN: transoral transpharyngeal approach to the brain. Neurosurg Rev 22:2-25

Resch KDM (2002) Postmortalinspection (PMI) for neurosurgery: a training model for endoscopic dissection technique. Neurosurg Rev 25:79-88

Resch KDM (2003) Endo-neuro-sonography (ENS). First clinical serie (52 cases). Childs Nerv Syst 19:137-144

Resch KDM, Perneczky A (1993) Endoscopic approaches to the suprasellar region: anatomy and current clinical applications. (Advances in neurosurgery, vol 22) Springer, Berlin Heidelberg New York

Resch KDM, Perneczky A (1994) Endoneurosurgery: anatomical basics. In: Samii M (ed) Skull base surgery. Karger, Basel

Resch KDM, Perneczky A (1997) Endo-neuro-sonography: anatomical aspects of the basal cisterns. Minim Invasiv Ther Allied Technol 6:332-339

Resch KDM, Perneczky A (1998) Endo-neuro-sonography: basics and current use. In: Hellwig D, Bauer BL (eds) Minimally invasive techniques for neurosurgery. Springer, Berlin Heidelberg New York, pp 21-31

Resch KDM, Reisch R (1997) Endo-neuro-sonography: anatomical aspects of the ventricles. Minim Invasive Neurosurg 1:2-7

Resch KDM, Perneczky A, Tschabitscher M, Kindel S (1994) Endoscopic anatomy of the ventricles. Acta Neurochir Suppl 61

Resch KDM, Reisch R, Hertel F, Perneczky A (1996) Endo-neuro-sonographie: eine neue Bildgebung in der Neurochirurgie. Endoskopie Heute 2(3) [whole issue]

Resch KDM, Hopf N, Kessel G, Perneczky A (1997a) Endo-neuro- sonography: new imaging technique in neurosurgery. Proceedings of the 11th International Congress of Neurological Surgery, Amsterdam, 6–11 June 1997, pp 1969-1974

Resch KDM, Atzor KR, Perneczky A (1997b) Anatomical phantom CT study of surgical approaches for 3-D and VR in neurosurgery. Minim Invasive Ther Allied Technol 6:228-234

Resch KDM, Perneczky A, Schwarz M, Voth D (1997c) Endo-neuro-sonography: principles and 3D technique. Childs Nerv Syst 13:616-621

Rieger A, Rainov NG, Sanchin L, Schopp G, Burkert W (1996) Ultrasound-guided endoscopic fenestration of the third ventricular floor for non-communicating hydrocephalus. Minim Invasive Neurosurg 39:17-20

Roelandt JRTC, ten Cater FJ, Brunning N et al (1993) Transoesophageal rotoplane echo-CT. A novel approach to dynamic three-dimensional echocardiography. The Thoraxcentre Journal 6(1) [whole issue]

Roelandt JRTC, ten Cater FJ, Vletter WB et al (1994) Ultrasonic dynamic three-dimensional visualization of the heart with a multiplane transoesophageal imaging transducer. J Am Soc Echocardiogr 7(3):217-229

Rosenfield K, Losordo DW, Ramaswamy K et al (1991) Three-dimensional reconstruction of human coronary and peripheral arteries from images recorded during two-dimensional intravascular ultrasound examination Circulation 84(5):1938-1956

Roth G (1999) Das Gehirn und seine Wirklichkeit. Surkamp, Frankfurt/Main, pp 258-311

Sacks O (1989a) Der Tag an dem mein Bein fortging. Rowohlt, Reinbek bei Hamburg, pp 205-222

Sacks O (1989b) Stumme Stimmen. Rowohlt, Reinbek near Hamburg, pp 117-182

Schlöndorf G (1998) Idee und Entwicklung der „Computer Assisted Surgery" an der RWTH in Aachen. Aachener Workshop on Navigierte Hirnchirurgie, Aachen, 4–5 September 1998, abstract book pp 1-3

Scholz M, Tombrock S, Konen W et al. (2005) Application of a newly developed visual navigation system in humans. First Results. Minim Invas Neurosurg 48:67-72

Schroeder HWS, Warzok RW, Assaf JA, Gaab MR (1999) Fatal subarachnoidal hemorrhage after endoscopic third ventriculostomy (case report). J Neurosurg 90:153-155

Schroeder HWS (2001) Historische Entwicklung der endoskopischen Neurochirurgie. In: Grumme T (ed) Neurochirurgie in Deutschland. Blackwell Wissenschaft, Berlin Vienna

Schroeder HWS, Gaab MR (1998) endoscopic management of intracranial arachnoid cysts. In: Hellwig D, Bauer LB (eds) Minimally invasive techniques for neurosurgery. Springer, Berlin Heidelberg New York

Schwartz S, Cao Q, Azevedo J, Pandian NG (1994) Simulation of intraoperative visualization of cardiac structures and study of dynamic surgical anatomy with real-time three-dimensional echocardiography. Am J Cardiol 73:501-507

Shekhar LN (2000) Comment: In: Paleologos TS, Wadley JP, Kitchen ND, Thomas GGT (2000) Clinical utility and cost-effectiveness of intracranial image-guided craniotomy: clinical comparison between conventional and image-guided meningioma surgery. Neurosurgery 47:40-48

Slovis TL, Canady A, Touchette A, Goldstein A (1991) Transcranial sonography through the burr hole for detection of ventriculomegaly. A preliminary report. J Ultrasound Med 10(4):195-200

Steinmeier R, Fahlbusch R, Ganslandt O et al (1998) Intraopertive magnetic resonance imaging with the Magnetome open scanner: concepts, neurosurgical indications, and procedures: a preliminary report. Neurosurgery 43:739-748

Strowitzki M, Ultrasound in Neurosurgery Study Group (2000) Ultraschall in der Neurochirurgie (abstract). Zentralbl Neurochir Suppl 1:6

Suhm N, Dams J, van Leyen K, Lorenz A, Bendl R (1998) Limitations for three-dimensional ultrasound imaging through burr hole trepanation. Ultrasound Med Biol 24(5):663-671

Sutcliffe JC (1991) The value of intraoperative ultrasound in neurosurgery. Br J Neurosurg 5(2):169-178

Taniguchi M, Takimoto H, Yoshimine T et al (1999) Application of rigid endoscope to the microsurgical management of 54 cerebral aneurysms: results in 48 patients. J Neurosurg 91:231-237

Tisell M, Almström O, Stephensen H, Tullberg M, Wikkelsö C (2000) How effective is endoscopic third ventriculostomy in treating adult hydrocephalus caused by primary aqueductal stenosis? Neurosurgery 46:104-109

Tronnier V, Staubert A, Wirtz R et al (1999) MRI-guided brain biopsies using 0.2 Tesla open magnet. Minim Invasive Neurosurg 42:118-122

Tsutsumi Y, Andoh Y, Sakaguchi J (1989) A new ultrasound-guided brain biopsy technique through a burr hole (technical note). Acta Neurochir (Wien) 96(1-2): 72-75

Van Roost D, Clusmann H, Urbach H, Helmstaedt C, Schramm J (2001) Transcortical versus transsylvian approach for selective amygdalo-hippocampectomy. 52nd Annual Meeting of the German Society of Neurosurgery, 27–30 May 2001, Bielefeld, abstract book, p 50

Van Velthoven V, Auer L M (1990) Practical application of intraoperative ultrasound imaging. Acta Neurochir (Wien) 105(1-2):5-13

Weinberg R (1992) Future direction in neurosurgery visualization. In: Apuzzo MLJ (ed) Neurosurgery for the Third Millennium. American Association of Neurological Surgeons, USA, pp 47-64

Weizäcker von V (1950) Der Gestaltkreis. Thieme, Stuttgart

Wickham J E (1993) Treatment of urinary tract stones. BMJ 307:1414-1417

Wirtz CR, Kunze S (1998) Neuronavigation: computerassistierte Neurochirurgie. Dtsch Arztebl 95:A-2384-2390

Wirtz CR, Tronnier VM, Bonsanto MM et al (1997) Image-guided neurosurgery with intraoperative MPI: updated frameless stereotaxy and radicality control. Stereotact Funct Neurosurg 68:39-43

Wirtz CR, Knauth M, Staubert A et al (2000) Clinical evaluation and follow-up results for intraoperative magnetic resonance imaging in neurosurgery. Neurosurgery 46:1112-1120

Wurm G, Wies W, Schnizer M, Trenkler J, Holl K (2000) Advanced surgical approach for selective amygdalo-hippocampectomy through neuronavigation. Neurosurgery 46:1377-1382

Yamakawa K, Kondo K, Yoshioka M, Takakura K (1994) Ultrasound guided endoscopic neurosurgery-new surgical instrument and technique. Acta Neurochir (Wien) Suppl 61:46-48

Yasargil MG (1969) Microsurgery applied to neurosurgery. Thieme, Stuttgart

Yasargil MG (1984a) Microneurosurgery, vol 1. Thieme, Stuttgart

Yasargil MG (1984b) Microneurosurgery, vol II. Thieme, Stuttgart New York

Yasargil MG (1994a) Microneurosurgery, vol IVA: Neuroradiology, conclusion. Thieme, Stuttgart, p 209

Yasargil MG (1994b) Microneurosurgery, vol IVA: CNS tumors: surgical anatomy, neuropathology, neuroradiology, neurophysiology, clinical considerations, operability, treatment options. Thieme, Stuttgart New York

Yasargil MG (1994c) Microneurosurgery, vol IVB: CNS tumors. Thieme, Stuttgart New York

Zorzic C, Angonese I (1989) Subependymal pseudocysts in the neonate. Eur J Pediatr 148(5):462-464

Subject Index

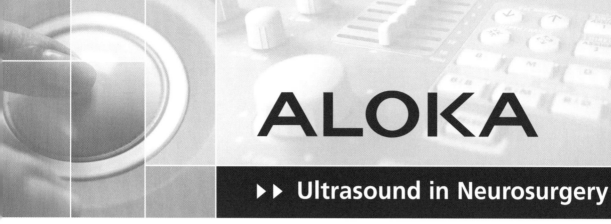
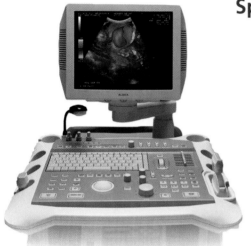
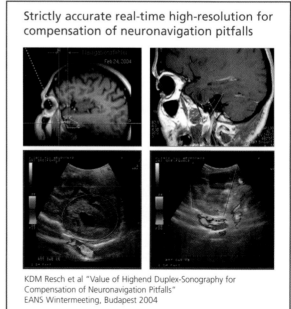
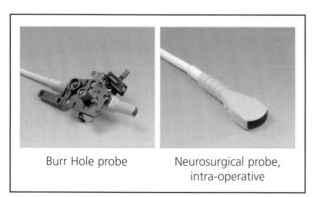

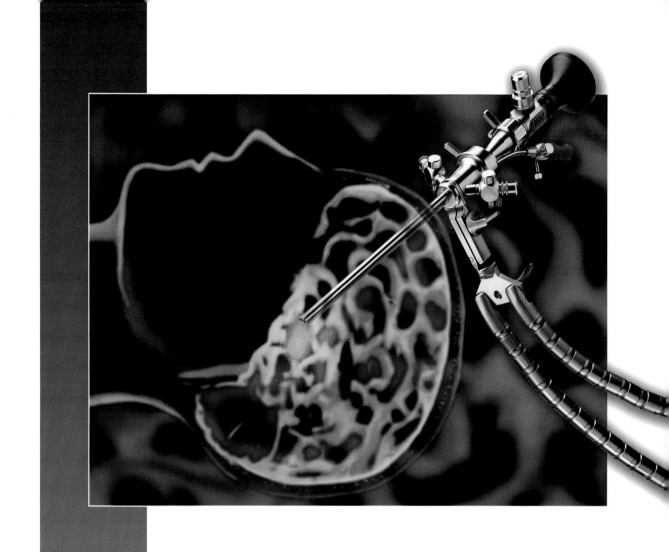

Neuroendoscopic Surgery Systems by Richard WOLF

- ❏ Pediatric Neuroendoscope System by Hopf
- ❏ Endoscopic Neurosurgery by Caemaert
- ❏ EANS System - Endoscopic Assisted Neuro Surgery

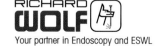

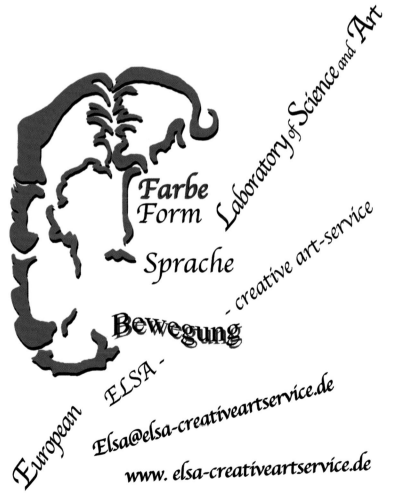

Farbe
Form

Laboratory of Science and Art

Sprache

- creative art-service

Bewegung

European   ELSA -

Elsa@elsa-creativeartservice.de

www. elsa-creativeartservice.de

extraordinary direct services in special fields of science and arts

Training Course on
Endo - Neuro - Sonography

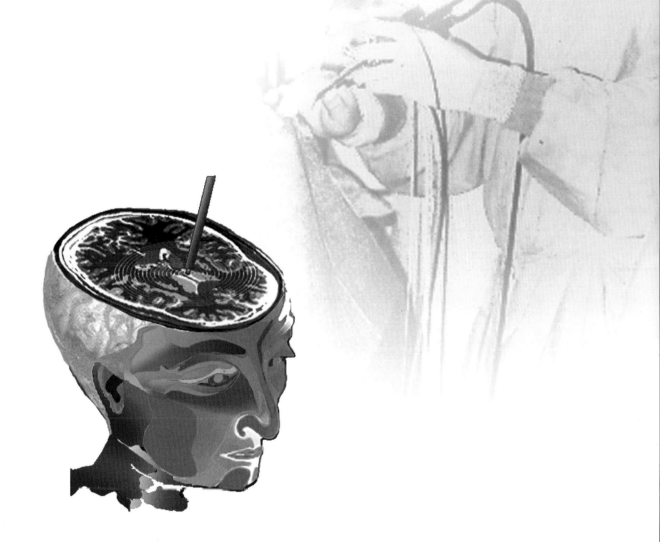

http://www.elsa-creativeartservice.de/science/ens.html